Ehsan Mamaghanizadeh
Haniyeh Bazavar
Zahra Yekanipour

Genetics

Ehsan Mamaghanizadeh
Haniyeh Bazavar
Zahra Yekanipour

Genetics

Noor Publishing

Imprint
Any brand names and product names mentioned in this book are subject to trademark, brand or patent protection and are trademarks or registered trademarks of their respective holders. The use of brand names, product names, common names, trade names, product descriptions etc. even without a particular marking in this work is in no way to be construed to mean that such names may be regarded as unrestricted in respect of trademark and brand protection legislation and could thus be used by anyone.

Cover image: www.ingimage.com

Publisher:
Noor Publishing
is a trademark of
Dodo Books Indian Ocean Ltd. and OmniScriptum S.R.L publishing group

120 High Road, East Finchley, London, N2 9ED, United Kingdom
Str. Armeneasca 28/1, office 1, Chisinau MD-2012, Republic of Moldova, Europe
Printed at: see last page
ISBN: 978-620-4-72450-8

Genetics

By

Ehsan Mamaghanizadeh

Department of Bacteriology and Virology, Faculty of Medical Sciences, Tabriz University of Medical Sciences, Tabriz, Iran

Haniyeh Bazavar

Department of Bacteriology and Virology, Faculty of Medical Sciences, Tabriz University of Medical Sciences, Tabriz, Iran

Zahra Yekanipour

Research Center for Clinical Virology, Tehran University of Medical Sciences, Tehran, Iran

Ehsan Mamaghanizadeh

Department of Bacteriology and Virology, Faculty of Medical Sciences, Tabriz University of Medical Sciences, Tabriz, Iran

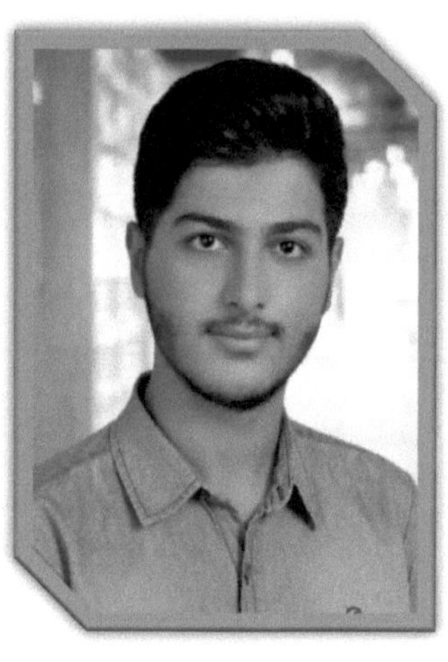

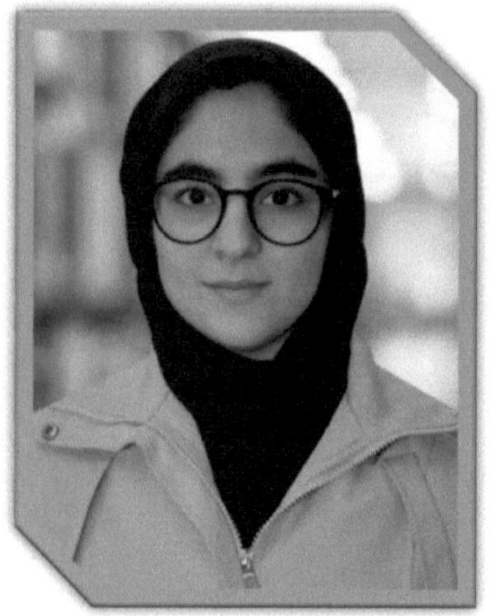

Haniyeh Bazavar

Department of Bacteriology and Virology, Faculty of Medical Sciences, Tabriz University of Medical Sciences, Tabriz, Iran

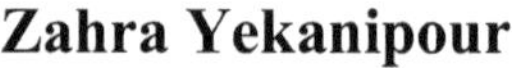

Zahra Yekanipour

Research Center for Clinical Virology, Tehran University of Medical Sciences, Tehran, Iran

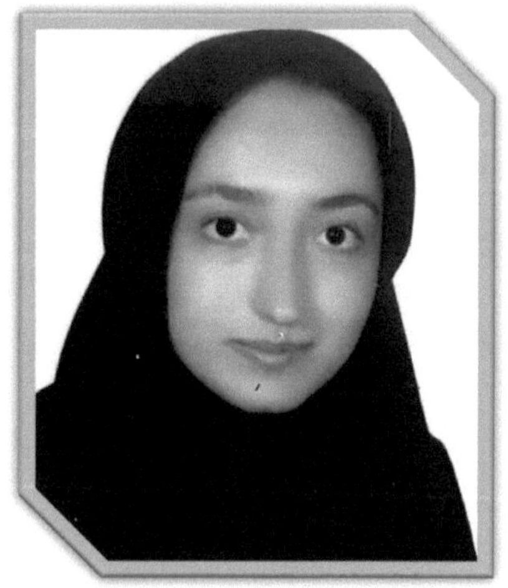

Dedicated to the merciful angels who:

The pure moments of believing, enjoying pleasure and pride, seeking courage, achieving greatness and all the unique and beautiful experiences of my life, are due to their green presence.

Dedication to my dear family.

Content

Chapter I

Introduction

Introduction

Genetics is a branch of biology that deals with the study of genes, genetic changes and inheritance in living organisms. Mendel studied the inheritance of traits, which is a model of how traits are passed from parents to children. He observed that organisms inherit discrete units of traits. This term, which is still used today, is a somewhat vague definition of what is referred to as a gene.

Inheritance of traits and molecular genetic mechanisms of genes are still the main principles of genetics in the 21st century, but modern genetics has gone beyond inheritance to study the function and behavior of genes. Gene structure and function, diversity and distribution are studied in the text of the cell, organism and in the context of the population. Genetics has created various fields such as molecular genetics, epigenetics and population genetics.

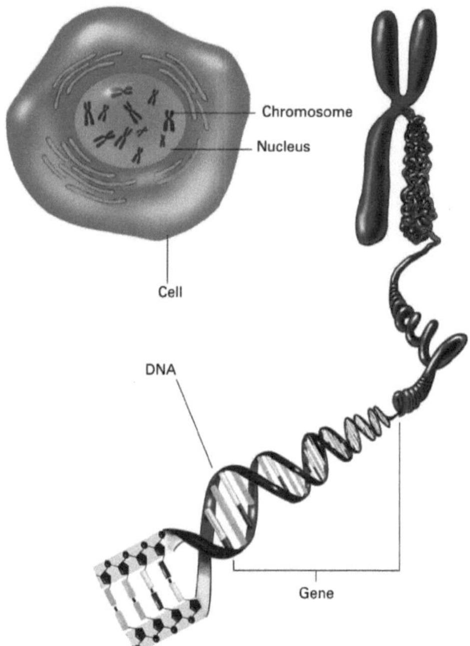

Figure 1. Genetics

The intracellular or extracellular environment of a living cell or organism may turn on or off the transcription of a gene. A classic example is two genetically similar maize grains, although one is in a temperate climate and the other is in a dry climate. For this reason, the average height of two corn stalks is genetically equal, but one in a dry climate grows only half the height of a corn stalk in a temperate climate due to the lack of water and nutrients in its environment.

Human genetic structure

For a better understanding of human genetic structure, we examine this structure from whole to part. There are 46 (23 pairs) chromosomes in the nucleus of each human cell, of which 22 pairs are asexual and one pair is sexual. According to the report of the correspondent of Servis Naghe blogs of Isna, he writes: each chromosome consists of a double-stranded DNA chain covered by special proteins. each DNA chain is formed from a sequence of organic bases. There are only four types of organic bases in each DNA strand, namely adenine (A), guanine (G), cytosine (C) and thymine (T). In two opposite strands in a DNA molecule, these bases are paired together.

Thymine is always in front of adenine and cytosine is always in front of guanine. Each gene, which is the unit of heredity, is a piece of DNA, that is, each gene is a specific sequence of organic base pairs. As mentioned, only four forms of organic base bond can be imagined, namely A-T, T-A, G-C and C-G. This limited number cannot justify countless genetic secrets, but when we know that each gene can contain thousands of organic base pairs and each DNA has approximately 3 billion organic base pairs, the matter will become clear. In each gene, all three organic base pairs act like a word that, when placed next to other words, make the genetic code that will eventually lead to the construction of an amino acid molecule.

These amino acids, in turn, will be responsible for the construction of thousands of proteins, including enzymes, which play a role in the formation and regulation of body functions, and based on the genetic instructions, some cells will become nerve cells and some will become eye lenses. They turn into heart valves and finally into a human being with unique characteristics. About 100,000 genes have been identified in each human. The human genome project, which is responsible for identifying the complete human genetic map, is supposed to be completed by 2005. Human genetic structure can be compared to a book. Suppose this book has 23 chapters called chromosomes and each chapter contains thousands of stories called genes. Each story is made up of paragraphs, and each paragraph is made up of words called codons, and each word is made up of letters called organic bases.

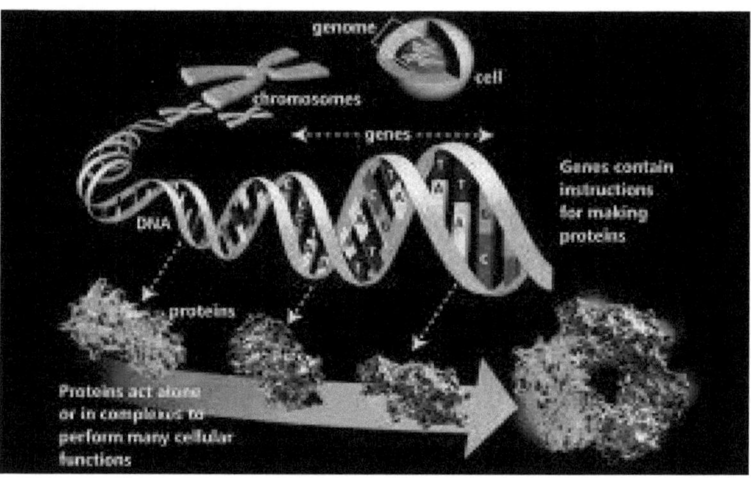

Figure 2. Genetics Basics

If we read the book of human genome at the speed of each word in one second, we need a century to finish it, and if we line up each letter one millimeter apart, it will be 1200 kilometers long. Chromosomes are in pairs in the cell nucleus. Therefore, each gene on one chromosome forms a pair of genes with its opposite gene on the other chromosome.

When a gene is called dominant when its effect appears on both homozygous and heterozygous people, it is called recessive when its effect is only on homozygous people. Sometimes, a specific trait in humans is the product of several genes acting simultaneously and together, which are referred to as multiple genes. Examples of traits that are controlled by several genes include skin color, height, weight, life span, degree of resistance to diseases, arterial blood pressure, and heart rate. These genes may occupy different positions on the chromosomes.

Some of them may be widely scattered on different pairs of chromosomes. The amount of a specific genetic trait that appears in a specific person is called gene penetration. Genes are usually fixed, but sometimes normal genes turn into abnormal genes. This change is called mutation. Mutation is one of the regular phenomena of nature and the number of natural mutations increases when exposed to mutagens such as ultraviolet rays, radiation and chemical carcinogens. Genotype and Phenotype Genotype refers to the entire genetic structure of each individual and phenotype refers to the external manifestations of this genetic structure.

Genotype is determined at the time of egg formation and remains constant throughout life, but phenotype may change from embryo to adulthood, such as height, weight, muscle mass, body shape. Therefore, genotype is the unchangeable aspect and phenotype is the changeable aspect of human genetic material. The genetic material can be compared to a piece of clay, the weight, volume, consistency and chemical properties of this piece of clay are fixed, but the potter can make it into different shapes. Therefore, it is said that medicine is the science of managing the human phenotype. Cell division is divided into two types: mitosis and meiosis. Mitosis is a type of cell division during which each cell chromosome is divided into two sister chromosomes called chromatids, and each of them goes to one of the daughter cells. During this process, each daughter cell will have exactly the same amount and the same type of sister chromosomes.

This type of division happens in all cells except sex cells. Germ cells reproduce through meiosis. Meiosis occurs in two cell divisions and only one chromosomal division. This form of division is also called reduced division. The result of this division is celling whose number of chromosomes is half of the original cell's chromosomes. This type of division happens in human sex cells.

Molecular genetics

Although genes were contained in chromosomes, chromosomes are composed of protein and DNA. For this reason, scientists do not know which of these two factors is heredity. In 1928, Frederick Griffith discovered the metamorphosis phenomenon. Sixteen years later, in 1944, the Avery-MacLeod-McCarty experiment identified DNA as the molecule responsible for transformation.

The Hershey-Chase experiment in 1952 confirmed that DNA is the genetic material of viruses that infect bacteria, providing further evidence that DNA is the molecule responsible for inheritance. James Watson and Francis crick determined the structure of DNA using X-ray crystallography. Rosalind franklin and Maurice Wilkins showed that DNA has a helical structure. This structure showed that genetic information is contained in the sequence of nucleotides in each strand of DNA.

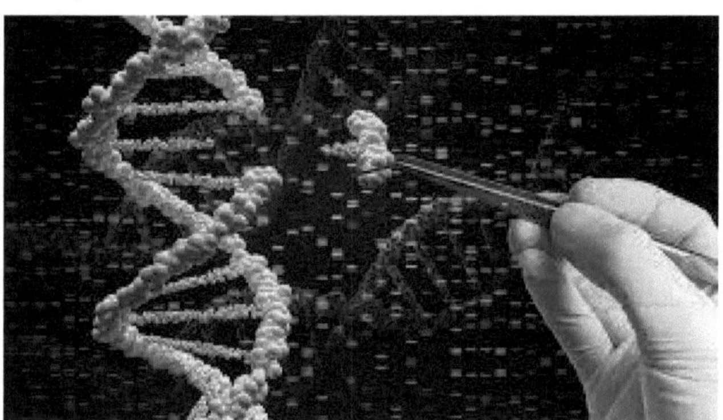

Figure 3. The Genetic Revolution

This structure also offers a simple method of reproduction. If strands diverge, new daughter strands can be rebuilt for each based on the sequence of the old strand. This property is what gives DNA its semi-conservative nature, where a new DNA strand is made from the parent strand. In recent years, scientists have tried to understand how DNA controls the process of protein production.

What is DNA?

DNA or deoxyribonucleic acid is the hereditary material in humans and almost all other organisms. Almost all cells in the body have the same DNA. Most DNA is located in the nucleus of the cell, but a small amount of DNA can also be found in the mitochondria. Mitochondria are structures inside cells that convert energy from food into a form that cells can use. The information in DNA is stored as a code made of four chemical bases adenine (A), guanine (G), cytosine (C) and thymine (T). Human DNA consists of about 3 billion bases, and more than 99% of these bases are the same in all people. The arrangement of these bases determines the information available to build and maintain the organism, similar to how the letters of the alphabet appear in a certain order to form words and sentences.

All about genetics

DNA bases pair with each other A with T and C with G to form units called base pairs. Each base also attaches to a sugar molecule and a phosphate molecule. These means a sugar and phosphate base together are called nucleotides. Nucleotides are arranged in two long strands that form a helix called a double helix. The structure of the double helix is almost like a ladder, with base pairs forming the rungs of the ladder, and sugar and phosphate molecules forming the main parts of the ladder. One of the important features of DNA is that it can replicate or make copies of itself. Each strand of DNA in the double helix can serve as a template for replicating a sequence of bases, which is critical in cell division. Because each new cell needs an exact copy of the DNA in the old cell.

What is a gene?

Gene is the main physical and functional unit of heredity. Genes are made of DNA. Some genes act as instructions for making molecules called proteins. However, many genes do not code for proteins. In humans, genes vary from a few hundred DNA bases to more than 2 million bases. The Human Genome Project estimates that humans have between 20,000 and 25,000 genes. Each person has two copies of each gene, one of which is inherited from each parent. Most genes are the same in all people, but a few genes differ slightly between people. Scientists track genes by giving them unique names. Because gene names can be long, genes are also assigned symbols, which are short combinations of letters that represent an abbreviated version of the gene name.

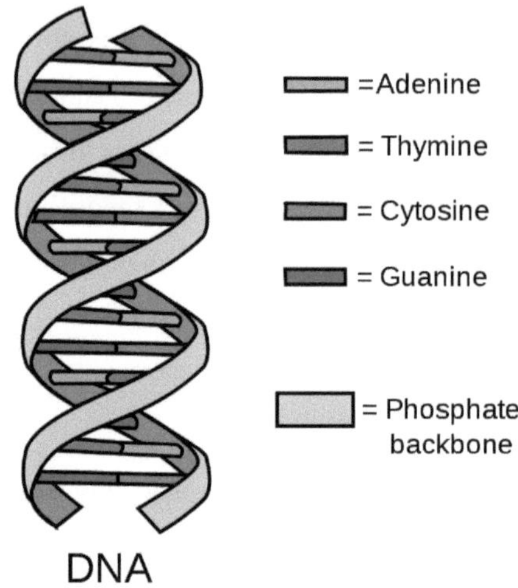

Figure 4. Building Blocks of the Genetic Code

What is a chromosome?

In the nucleus of each cell, DNA molecules are packaged into thread-like structures called chromosomes. Each chromosome is made of DNA that is tightly wrapped multiple times around proteins called histones that support its structure. Chromosomes in the nucleus of the cell are not visible even under a microscope during cell division. However, the DNA that makes up the chromosomes becomes more tightly packed during cell division and is then visible under a microscope.

Most of what researchers know about chromosomes has been learned by observing chromosomes during cell division. Each chromosome has a contraction point called a centromere, which divides the chromosome into two parts or arms. The short arm of the chromosome is called the p arm and the long arm is called the q arm. The location of the centromere of each chromosome gives the chromosome a specific shape and can be used to describe the location of specific genes.

How many chromosomes do humans have?

In humans, each cell normally has 23 pairs of chromosomes. Twenty-two of these pairs, called autosomes, are the same in both males and females. The 23 pairs of sex chromosomes are different between men and women. Females have two copies of the X chromosome, while males have one X and one Y chromosome. This picture of human chromosomes that are in pairs is called karyotype.

Genetic laboratories and clinics

Before the development of modern genetic technologies, genetic services were limited to genetic counseling, where health professionals attempted to describe the genetic contribution of diseases based on family history. With the discovery of DNA, genetic services have increased dramatically in quality and scope.

Today, advanced technologies using new methods and high-quality preparations allow greater accuracy in diagnosis. Today, the presence of genetic laboratories and clinics around the world is significant. Many hospitals with established genetics programs offer specialized laboratory and comprehensive diagnostic evaluation in addition to genetic counseling. In the absence of an expert genetic counselor, nurses and other health care workers are often trained to counsel patients.

In addition to the work of independent genetic researchers, laboratories and clinics also address the needs and services of the public. These include the identification of mutations to the analysis of susceptibility to disease, the identification of diseases in the unborn fetus, in addition to explaining the possible risks caused by genetic influences in pregnancies and methods of their prevention.

History of genetics

To know the truth of what happened in the past, one must search in more than one scientific source. We all know the science of genetics by the name of the Austrian monk scientist Mr. Gregor Mendel, the father of genetics, but did Mendel initiate continuous efforts to discover the endless world of genes? The answer to this question is negative. In 1866, he started his work with his possible theories and during his research, he sought help from the information of his predecessors.

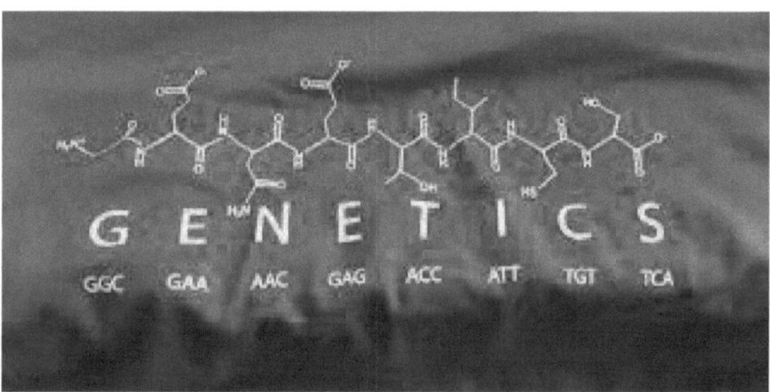

Figure 5. UW, Madison Genetics

From Pythagoras to Mendel

The history of genetics starts from the classical era with the participation of Pythagoras, Hippocrates, Aristotle, Epicurus and other ancient scientists. In the following, we will explain the theory of these scientists about genetics and the inheritance of traits:

1- **Hippocrates' genetic theory:** the first writings related to the subject of heredity are related to Hippocrates, a Greek physician and the so-called father of western medicine and Aristotle. The theory of Hippocrates is known as the brick-and-mortar genetic theory and says that taxonomic materials include physical materials that originate from all parts of the body and accumulate in men's semen, and these materials turn into a human being inside the woman's womb.

2- Aristotle and opposition to Hippocrates' theory: According to reports in the history of genetics, Aristotle did not agree with Hippocrates' brick and mortar theory. Because he believed that this theory cannot explain heredity in areas of the body such as nails, hair, voice. Because these traits are caused by dead tissues and cannot play a role in reproduction. Aristotle also pointed out that children may be more like their grandparents than their parents, and therefore the substances involved in reproduction are not collected from different parts of the body, but rather they are nutrients that are used in order to Reproduction has been created and specialized. Aristotle also believed that women also play a role in determining the shape and some characteristics of the fetus.

3- Pythagoras and genetics: Pythagoras of Samos was an ancient Greek philosopher and the famous founder of Pythagoreanism. Pythagoras thought that all the hereditary characteristics are passed from the father to the child and the mother only provides the place and nutrition of the fetus. He believed that semen is a combination of hereditary information that travels through a man's body, collecting fluids in every organ on its travels. Finally, when the man pours it inside the woman's vagina, these liquid forms a child in the mother's womb.

4- Epicurus and dominant and dominant inheritance: In the reports in the history of medicine, it is stated that the Athenian philosopher Epicurus realized the role of men and women in creating hereditary characteristics by observing families. He also paid attention to the types of dominant and recessive inheritance models and separated and introduced the independent set of sperm atoms.

History of genetics

The origins and history of modern genetics can be traced back to Gregor Mendel's memoirs about the hybridization of the pea plant in 1865 by fertilizing pea plants and examining their second and third generations after fertilization, Mendel realized that there are special rules for the transmission of traits. However, the word genetics was coined in 1906 to denote the new science and information of heredity. This science, which is based on the Mendelian method for the analysis of heredity, explains concepts such as genes, genotypes and phenotypes. However, Mendel's theories were not supported by scientific societies until after his death. He has three important laws called Mendel's laws, which are:

The first law: the law of segregation of genes.

The second law: the law of independent matching of genes.

The third law: the law of predominance.

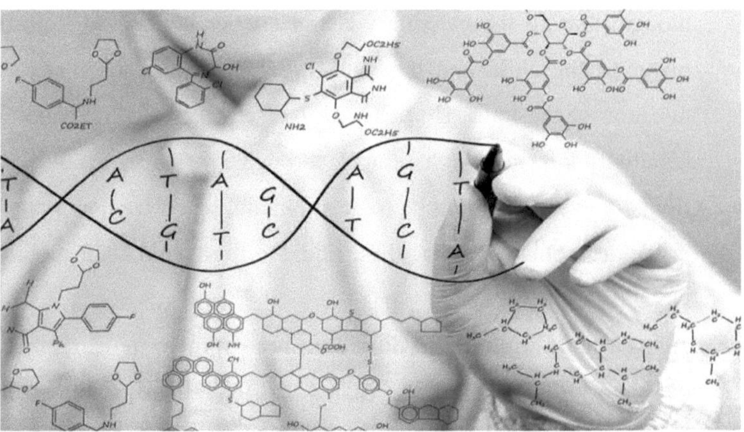

Figure 6. Online Genetics Course, 100% Online Science Prerequisite

Drevis's efforts for modern genetics

In 1900, new discoveries made the laws presented by Gregor Mendel to be noticed and accepted by scientists such as Dervis, Shermak and Cornes, and finally Mendel was called the father of genetics by the scientific community. These few scientists, led by

Thomas Hunt Morgan, developed Mendelian laws, which were widely accepted by researchers in 1925. With the introduction of the basic patterns of genetic inheritance, many biologists turned to investigate the physical nature of genes, so that in the 1940s and early 1950s, the results of experiments and research on DNA as a part of chromosomes that hold genes, they remembered the focus on other organisms such as viruses and bacteria along with the discovery of the helical structure of DNA in 1953 marked the transition to the era of molecular genetics.

In the following years, chemists developed techniques for sequencing nucleic acids and proteins, determined the relationship between these two forms of biological molecules, and discovered the genetic code. The regulation of gene expression became a major topic in the 1960s, and during the 1970s gene expression was controlled and manipulated by basic science researchers through genetic engineering. In the last decades of the 20th century, many biologists focused on large-scale genetic projects, such as sequencing whole genomes, and achieved surprising results. This fundamental discovery that the cell is the basic unit of all living organisms took place relatively late in the history of human life. In 1677, a Dutch scientist named Van Leeuwenhoek, whose hobby was making simple microscopes, managed to be the first person to observe microbial objects, including bacteria.

In 1838, a German botanist named Matthias Schleiden, after looking at plant tissues with the more powerful microscopes of that time, proposed the idea that plants are made of simple units called cells. Shortly after that time, a German zoologist named Theodor Schwann made a similar proposal to the theory of Matthias Schleiden for animals. It took 20 years for the cell structure to be accepted for all living organisms. The German pathologist, Rudolph Wiershaw, expressed this cell theory at least about animals in this way: every animal is a collection of vital units, each of which contains the complete characteristics of life.

Therefore, it became clear that understanding the basis of life is necessary to understand how the cell is structured and how it works. Determining the two types of cells, especially the egg and sperm cells, was the basis of the understanding of the heir. Egg and sperm are both necessary for the beginning of every human life. Sperm is a cell that is specialized for swimming and does not have many components except the structures necessary for swimming and a nucleus, hence the assumption that the nucleus of the cell plays an important role in the creation of new human life.

In 1879, a German biologist named Walter Fleming, using a microscope, succeeded in observing that the small particles inside the cell nucleus, which they call chromosomes, have doubled. It took another 20 years for an American scientist named Walter Sutton to observe in 1903 that during gamete formation, each gamete receives only one of the pairs of chromosomes in the gamete-producing cell. Gametes in humans, eggs and sperm are special cells that are used in sexual reproduction.

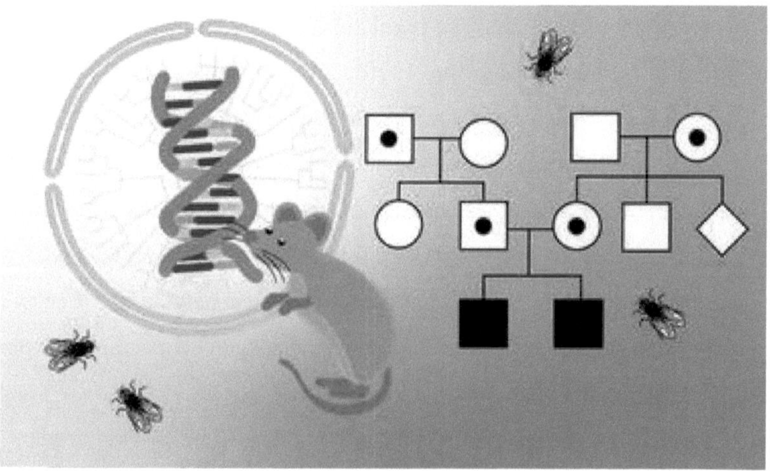

Figure 7. Genetics: The Fundamentals

As a result, Sutton proposed that this order must have a fundamental cause and suggested that the genetic information is inserted in a special way and place on the chromosome. Sutton's proposal was based not only on his own findings, but also on Gregor Mendel's discoveries, which he had observed in practice 40 years before Sutton. Mendel claimed that the traits observed in the pea plant are determined by factors that are paired with each other and we call them genes today. Each parent transmits only one of each pair of factors to its offspring. Sutton's proposal that inheritance is chromosomal, combined genetics with molecular biology, the former of which proposed the existence of genes, but did not pay attention to their material basis, and the latter observed cellular order and nuclear division, but compared to the structures observed in the active cell.

Why do children resemble their parents?

People must have asked themselves this question for thousands of years. The first written answer to this question is found in a book attributed to the Greek physician Hippocrates. According to Hippocrates, semen contains the characteristics of everybody that produced it, but Aristotle rejected this opinion with the argument that, for example, the children of crippled people do not necessarily inherit these defects. Aristotle instead suggested that semen teaches the mother how to make a child? As, for example, a carpenter is told how to make a table from pieces of wood.

Therefore, Aristotle presented a very new idea, that is, seminal fluid contains information, but this idea was forgotten by the generations after him. There are very few references to inheritance in medieval writings. In 1660, the Italian physiologist Marcello Malpighi proposed that the human ovum cell contains a very small preform called a dummy, which the mother received from her mother and her mother received from her mother, and based on this analogy, this Chinese box theory is the origin of dummies. traces it to Eve.

After Léon Hooke discovered in 1677 that seminal fluid contained sperm, the dummy was placed in the sperm instead of the egg. However, the dummy theory was problematic because it could not explain how it is possible for children to inherit some of their traits from the mother but others from the father. The first decisive experiments that led to the discovery of the laws of heredity were carried out by Gregor Mendel and the Austrian monk. Mendel published his theory in 1865. He knew that it is possible to change the color of ornamental flowers by mixing different plants with each other, and from such combinations, repeatable results can be obtained. Mendel was interested in understanding the principles underlying this phenomenon.

Mendel took his investigations of heredity further by mating pure plant samples that differed on several distinct traits. He found that the inheritance of each trait is independent of the inheritance of other traits. In this way, Mendel discovered the principle of the independence of inheritance of different traits and strengthened the idea of the particle nature of genetic information. Mendel's findings remained buried in 120 libraries around the world for 35 years, without anyone realizing its value, until in 1900, three separate people, without knowing each other's work, the Dutch scientist Hugo de Vries, the German researcher Karl Cornes and the scientist Eric Chermak Austrians rediscovered Mendelian principles.

It wasn't long before the English scientist William Batson suggested that the study of heredity deserved a specific name and proposed the name genetics, which is derived from the Greek word meaning born or produced. Since then, the science of genetics has grown rapidly, but it is interesting that this science flourished for more than 50 years, without anyone knowing what a gene is. Despite this, a lot of inferential knowledge about the nature of genes and the organization of genes was provided by mixing organisms together and observing the phenotype of their offspring.

In 1908, Thomas Morgan, an American geneticist, started using Drosophila in genetic research. The main advantages of using Drosophila are that it reproduces quickly, so that the duration of creating a generation is only three weeks, and the offsprings obtained from a single mating reach 100. The size of this fly is small and its population needs a small space and its feeding costs little.

The first mutant flies that Morgan obtained had white eyes instead of red, and Morgan's research showed that the mutant phenotype was inherited in a simple way. Morgan soon created large groups of Drosophila that differed in several traits. He found that while many combinations of traits are inherited independently of each other, some traits can also be inherited together. In fact, this is what Mendel had already proved, and Morgan called this phenomenon continuity.

These findings answer the question of what is a gene? They did not answer, but they suggest a lot of knowledge about the organization of genes. A breakthrough was made when genetic research using bacteria was expanded. The bacteria grow quickly, and experiments with them only take a few weeks instead of years. In 1928, Frederick Griffith, an English scientist, showed that it is possible to mix bacteria that were killed by heat with bacteria that have other characteristics to obtain bacteria that have the characteristics of both live and dead bacteria groups.

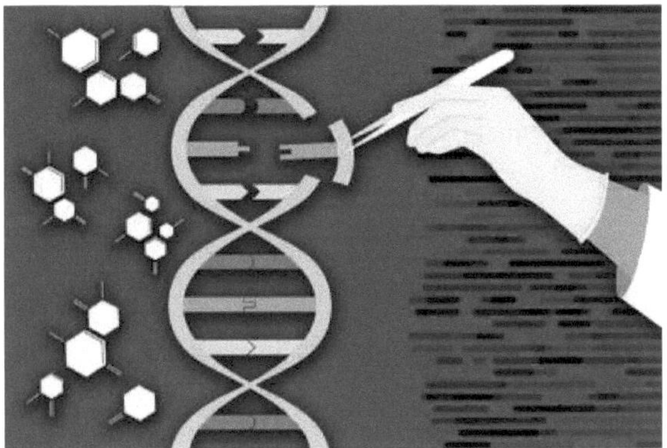

Figure 8. Genetics

This is the same phenomenon that he called transformation. Griffith's argument was that the dead bacteria must have given something to the living bacteria that changed their genetic makeup. In 1944, American geneticists Oswald Avery, Colin McLeod and MacLean McCarthy determined that the chemical was responsible for DNA transformation. This was the first empirical evidence to confirm that the chemical substance that was described in 1871 more than 70 years ago by Friedrich Miescher in Tübingen, contained the key to life, the gene.

It didn't take long to find out that the DNA molecule is very long and its structure is relatively uniform at first glance, consisting of only adenine, thymine, cytosine and guanine. In the DNA molecule of every living organism, there is a common feature, and that is the equality of the number of bases adenine with thymine and cytosine with guanine.

The combination of these facts with the knowledge of the structure of DNA obtained from the analysis of DNA crystal images by X-ray diffraction, together with the theoretical understanding of the structural conditions of the molecule carrying genetic information, led English scientist Francis Crick and American James Watson to work together in Cambridge, suggested that the structure of the DNA molecule is a double-stranded helix. This proposal was made in 1953, 53 years after the rediscovery of Mendelian laws, but Francis and Watson could not prove their hypothesis. At the same time, when these two scientists were engaged in research, other scientists named Morris Wilkins and Rosalin Fraklin had photographed the DNA molecule using X-ray radiation, but these two scientists themselves did not succeed in interpreting the content of the photo.

A view of Franklin's X-ray photograph of the DNA molecule

Maurice Wilkins was close friends with Francis and James Watson, and because of this, at a party to which all three were invited, Maurice showed Watson and Francis the photograph taken by Franklin, but he never knew that Francis and James had the same photograph. They will prove the ladder model of the DNA molecule. After looking at the photo, Frances and James asked Maurice to keep it on loan and Maurice gave it to them. Watson and Crick took the photo to their lab where they worked on it for almost 2 months and were finally able to interpret Franklin's photo of the DNA molecule, which resulted in the proof of the ladder model of the DNA molecule, but the two scientists never named Franklin.

They did not play the most important role in proving the ladder model of the DNA molecule. Rosaline Franklin died of cancer at the age of 38, but her memory will always be immortalized as one of the world's celebrities. Now the golden age of molecular biology had begun. How is it possible that a uniform molecule like DNA, that is, a molecule that consists of only four types of bases and therefore can encode information with only four letters at most, has the capacity to explain the structure of thousands of types of enzymes. It was known many years ago that every living organism has a large number of genes and a large number of enzymes.

The idea that many of these genes direct the production of enzymes was established in 1941 by two American geneticists, George Biddle and Edward Tatum, who were working with a type of mold called Neurosporacrassa. These two researchers showed that in some cases, the mutation of a mold gene prevented the growth of that mold, unless some kind of vitamin was added to its culture medium. They determined that this mutated mold behavior was the result of the loss of one of the enzymes necessary for the synthesis of that vitamin. This is why Biddle and Tatum proposed the one-gene-one-enzyme hypothesis, that is, each gene encodes the production of one enzyme. This hypothesis was formulated before the structure of DNA was determined. The structure of DNA clarified only two things.

First, it provided a mechanism for the replication of genetic material, that is, the double-stranded helix can determine the construction of two other DNA molecules whose structure is identical to the structure of the original DNA molecule. He also proposed the reason for the connection of genes, and that is if a long DNA molecule can contain enough information to match a number of genes, but the question of how DNA can guide the making of protein molecules remained unsolved.

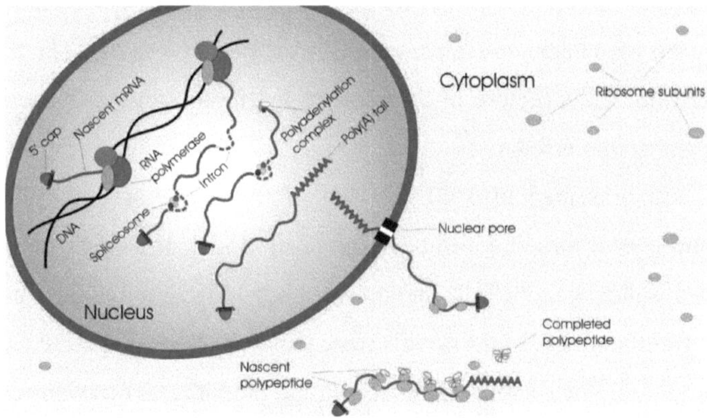

Figure 9. Genetic Mechanisms

As we know, protein is a long biomolecule made of 22 amino acids, and each protein molecule contains many amino acids. Three open molecules of DNA are needed to code each amino acid, and each of these triplets is called a codon or code. As a result of the research, the genetic code was read in several laboratories.

Great world celebrities in the science of genetics

The precise genetic experiments carried out in 1961 at the Laboratory of Molecular Genetics of the University of Cambridge made an important contribution to this success. These experiments were conducted by a group of scientists led by Sidney Brenner and Francis Crick. Crick had already proposed that there should be a type of peak that transfers the genetic information related to protein synthesis from the DNA inside the nucleus to the cytoplasm where the protein is made, and today it is known that this peak is the mRNA molecule.

François Jacob and Jacques Monad at the Institute Pasteur in Paris in 1961 suggested that the simple idea that genes produce proteins automatically and non-stop is not true, but that the application of genetic information is regulated and programmed. These two scientists proposed the operon model for gene structure and proposed that a gene or a group of genes is associated with a piece of DNA called a promoter. The trigger action is not to determine the structure of the protein, but to control the transcription of its neighboring genes into mRNA.

This model was presented in 1961 for one of the genes of the Escherichia coli bacterium, and later it turned out to be a universal model, at least in basic principles. In the mid-1960s, how genetic information was coded by DNA and their use in protein synthesis was well defined. Many details were still to be known, but the essence of the mystery was solved. The science of molecular and human genetics was advancing at a great speed.

Some geneticists also have medical knowledge, but in general, the medical world is slow to understand the importance of genetic science. Doctors at that time were not aware of the importance of genetic science for human health. Interestingly, almost 50 years have passed since the invention of techniques to observe chromosomes, but the exact number of chromosomes was not determined until 1956. In 1956, it was discovered that the first known abnormality, Down syndrome, was caused by having an abnormal number of chromosomes. It was probably this discovery that caused the medical world to gradually treat genetic science more seriously.

The major movement occurred in 1980 when it was discovered that viruses can induce cancer in humans.

From that moment on, the medical world's interest in genetic science gained an increasing speed. The gap between the first attempt at gene therapy in humans and the opening of the first gene therapy institute in March 1994 at the University of Pennsylvania was only four years. Even now, the science of genetics is advancing at a very fast pace.

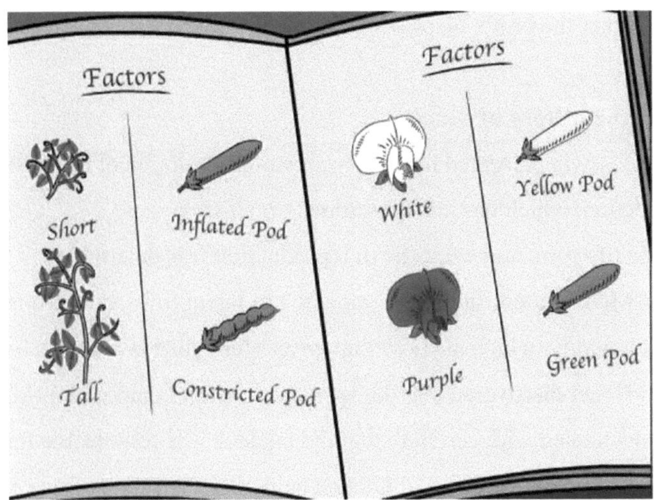

Figure 10. Genetics

Milestones in the history of cell theory

1665: Robert Hooke first described the cells he observed in cork.

1667: Van Leeuwenhoek observed and described bacteria and other microbes using a primitive microscope. At that time, many people believed that microbes were produced spontaneously.

1765: Spallanzani was the first to show that organisms do not arise spontaneously. He boiled a piece of meat with water and closed the lid of the container. The broth in the container remained clear. Proponents of spontaneity argued that the absence of air in a closed container prevented the growth of microbes in that container.

1838: Mathias Schleiden proposed after microscopic observations that plants are composed of units called cells.

1839: Theodor Schwann made a proposal similar to Schleiden's about animal tissues.

1858: Rudolf Virchow proposed a theory that became accepted as the cell theory. Every animal is a collection of vital units, each of which has all the characteristics of a living organism.

1864: Louis Pasteur repeated Spallanzani's experiment using a strong necked glass that allowed air to enter the broth, disproving the theory of spontaneous generation.

Milestones in the history of genetics

1859: Charles Darwin presented his theory about the evolution of organisms by means of natural selection, which has unified various organisms.

1860: The role of sperm and egg cells in reproduction was determined.

1865: Gregor Mendel identified the dominant and latent traits and also invented laws to understand heredity, which are now known as Mendelian laws.

1868: Eduard Hegel discovered that the sperm was a cell composed mostly of nuclear material and postulated with certainty that the nucleus was responsible for heredity.

1871: Frederic Miescher discovered nucleic acid, DNA, in the nucleus of cells taken from a pus wound.

1875: Hertog observed the fertilization of animals and accepted as a principle of certainty that each cell nucleus is derived from another nucleus.

1879: Walter Fleming described the duplication of chromosomes in the nucleus.

1900: Carl Korns together with Eric Chermack and Hugo Vries separately rediscovered Mendelian laws.

1903: Walter Sutton discovered that each gamete receives one of the two chromosomes from each pair of chromosomes present in a diploid cell.   He accepted as a principle of certainty that genetic information is contained in chromosomes.

1908: Thomas Morgan researched Drosophila and proved that the gene is the unit of hereditary information and can be changed by mutation.

1909: Walter Johansen popularized the name gene for the hereditary unit.

1927: Hermann Müller and Louis Stadler separately demonstrated that X-rays could induce mutations in Drosophila.

1941: George Biddle and Edward Tatum, by researching the mold Neurospora crassa, proposed as a certainty that each gene is responsible for the production of an enzyme.

1943: Luria and Delbork proved that the bacterium Escherichia coli can spontaneously become resistant to bacterial viruses. This discovery changed the face of genetic science and marked the beginning of the victory of Escherichia coli bacteria as the lifeblood of genetic research.

1944: Oswald Avery, Colin McLeod and McLean McCarthy resolved the long-standing scientific debate that DNA is the material of heredity by researching the bacterium Pneumococcus pneumoniae.

1945: Delbrook of the Phage School began the study of microbial parasite viruses in Cold Spring Harbor, USA, which had a tremendous impact on genetics and molecular biology.

1949: Eric Chargaff discovered that the adenine content of the DNA molecule is equal to its thymine content and its guanine content is equal to its cytosine content, but the amount of A+T in the DNA molecule of different species of organisms is different.

1950: Maurice Wilkins and Rosalyn Franklin obtained the first X-ray photographs of DNA, showing that DNA has an ordered structure.

1951: McLintock proved with corn research that some genes can move from one point to another in a chromosome.

1952: Hersky and Chips discovered that DNA is the genetic material of bacterial viruses. The number of those who were still in favor of the protein content of the genetic material was reduced.

1953: Francis Crick and James Watson interpreted Wilkins and Franklin's photographs of the DNA molecule and proposed a double helix structure for that molecule. These scientists proposed that this type of structure allows the DNA molecule to replicate in a very simple way.

1953: Luria, Yeoman, Bertani and Weigel discovered the phenomenon of restriction and modulation, which led to the discovery of restriction enzymes in molecular techniques.

1961: François Jacob and Jacques Monad proved that gene activity in E.coli should be regulated by external factors and proposed the first gene expression regulation model.

1970: Mitzotani, Baltimore and Temin discovered by researching viruses that the central principle of Francis Crick's proposal should be adjusted, there is an enzyme called reverse transcription enzyme or reverse transcriptase that can synthesize a double-stranded DNA molecule from a single-stranded RNA molecule.

1977: Roberts and Sharp discovered the existence of introns in eukaryotes.

1828: Wehler first synthesized urea, which is an organic molecule, in the laboratory. Urea is found in animal urine. This discovery showed that organic materials can be synthesized from inorganic materials.

1857: Louis Pasteur first demonstrated the enzymatic reaction in a microscopic organism. During wine fermentation, glucose is converted into ethanol in the yeast cell.

1897: Buchner was the first person to show the enzymatic reaction in the test tube that glucose is converted into ethanol by the extract of yeast cells in the absence of living cells.

1900: Fischer proposed that the amino acids of the protein molecule are connected by chemical bonds.

1926: George Sumner was the first to purify the urease enzyme that breaks down urea.

1949: Pauling proved that sickle cell anemia was caused by an abnormal hemoglobin molecule.

1949: Brecht and Casperson discovered that RNA is located in the cytoplasm of eukaryotic cells and is also the site of protein synthesis.

1953: Frederick Sanger determined the amino acid sequence of a type of protein called insulin for the first time. Today, Sanger sequencing is used in nucleotide sequence.

1956: Korenberg proved that the DNA molecule could be duplicated in a test tube.

1957: Ingram showed that the hemoglobin of patients with sickle cell anemia differs in only one amino acid from the hemoglobin of healthy individuals, and after the discovery of the genetic code, it became possible to observe that a change of just one nucleotide can make a person sick.

1956-58: Zemneck and Hoagland discover the adapter molecule hypothesized by Francis Crick, now called transfer RNA.

1965: Erber proved that the restriction phenomenon is caused by an enzyme that cuts DNA, but not precisely.

1970: Smith first isolated the restriction enzyme that cuts the DNA molecule at a very specific nucleotide.

The beginning of the era of genetic engineering

1973: Cohen and Bayer synthesized the first recombinant DNA.

1977: Maxam and Gilbert and Sanger discovered two different methods for DNA sequencing.

1983: Gary Mullis discovers the polymerase chain reaction (PCR) technique that converts a piece of DNA into millions of copies in a relatively short time.

1987: Smith made a gene mutate in a test dish and then reintroduced it back into a living cell.

Milestones in the history of human genetics

1900: Karl Landsteiner presented the ABO blood group system to mankind. With this great discovery, blood transfusion between humans became possible without risk and safety.

1902: Garo studied one of the human diseases, Alkaptonuria. The patient excretes homogenous acid in his urine, which is seen in dark color in the vicinity of air by studying the family trees of the patients' families, Garrow realized that the laws of inheritance discovered by Mendel provided a reasonable explanation for this phenomenon, which was consistent with the mode of inheritance of latent traits. Garo was the first to suggest the relationship between a genetic defect and the absence of an enzyme. Despite the fact that Garrow held an honorary chair of medicine at Oxford University, the value of his creative contribution to the science of human genetics remained unknown during his lifetime. Biologists did not pay much attention to the work of a doctor, and the medical world did not understand the importance of Garo's findings for medicine.

1911: Van Dungeren and Hirschfeld demonstrated the ABO mode of inheritance of the blood system, which is a striking example of the application of Mendelian inheritance to a human trait.

1911: Frederick Roos was the first to discover a virus that causes cancer in domestic animals or chickens, the Roos sarcoma virus.

1956: Tejo and Luan proved that humans have a total of 46 chromosomes.

1959: Legion reported that Down syndrome may be caused by having three copies of chromosome 21 instead of the normal two.

1965: Harris and Afroosi developed methods for fusing mouse and human cells. With this work, it became possible to determine the location of many genes in special chromosomes. Since then, other methods have been invented, and today, more than 23,000 human genes have been mapped that encode proteins with a known function.

1980: Bishop and Varmus proved that viruses can induce some types of cancer in humans.

1981: Wirgler first isolated a gene from humans that causes cancer when mutated.

1990: Blaise, Culver and French Anderson performed gene therapy for the first time at the National Institutes of Health in Bethesda, USA.

Since two hundred thousand years ago, when the first human civilization appeared on earth, until now, mankind has always tried to understand the secrets of life due to his inner curiosity towards everything that was unclear to him, and today the same techniques that It was invented by human hands, it has made the way of thinking easier and faster, and everything that was once vague and dumb for humans, has been put into practice today.

What is genetic testing?

Genetic testing is the laboratory analysis of the genetic material of the human body. This test includes chromosomes, deoxyribonucleic acid (DNA) or ribonucleic acid (RNA) to detect genetic material or identify genetic changes. Certain segments of DNA, called genes, serve as templates for making RNA. Genetic changes are referred to as changes and can have different effects on the body. Although most genetic changes do not affect a person's health, they are sometimes associated with disease.

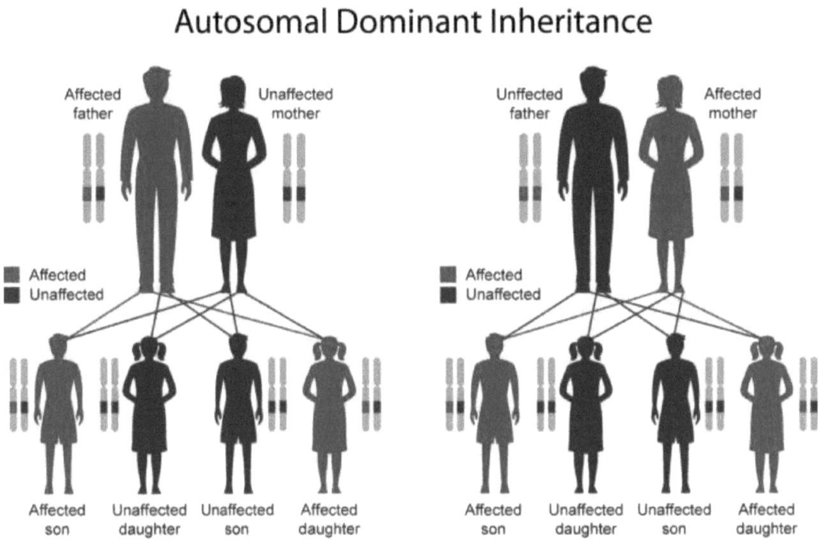

Autosomal Dominant Inheritance

Figure 11. Genetics and Inheritance

How is genetic testing done?

Some type of body sample is required for genetic testing. This sample can be blood, urine, saliva, body tissues, bone marrow, hair, etc. The sample can be received in a tube, on a swab, in a container or frozen. After that, the genetic material is separated and removed from the sample in a specialized laboratory. Some genetic disorders are linked to a single gene, and genetic testing typically focuses on testing for mutations in genes based on a person's symptoms or family history.

For example, cystic fibrosis has a well-defined set of symptoms, and testing for mutations in a single gene can usually identify the cause of these symptoms. However, there are many other genetic disorders that are not easily identified. These are linked to several genes or large parts of the genome. The following sections provide an overview of genetic testing methods, ranging from identifying or examining a single gene to the entire genome.

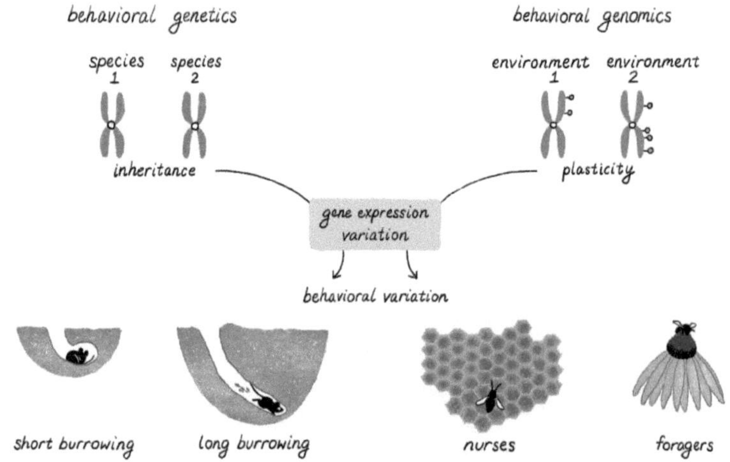

Figure 12. Behavioral genetics and genomics: Mendel's peas, mice, and bees

Chapter II

Genetic testing methods

❖ PCR method: PCR polymerase chain reaction is a common method for making the amplification of short segments of DNA from a very small sample of genetic material. This process is called DNA amplification and allows the genes or regions of interest to be identified or measured. This method is often used for DNA replication.

❖ DNA sequence: DNA sequence is determined by determining the order of the bases adenine (A), thymine (T), cytosine (C) and guanine (G) that make up DNA. Sequencing helps doctors determine whether a gene or the region that regulates a gene contains a change or changes.

❖ Cytogenetics (karyotype and FISH): Everyone has 23 pairs of chromosomes, including 22 pairs of autosomes and one pair of sex chromosomes. The science related to the study of these chromosomes is called cytogenetics. Trained cytogenetic specialists examine the number, shape and staining pattern of these structures using special technologies. In this way, they can detect extra chromosomes, missing chromosomes, or rearranged chromosomes.

❖ Microarrays: Microarray testing is a technique that is used for various purposes. Microarrays are used in diagnostic tests to determine whether a person's DNA contains duplications, deletions, or large stretches of the same DNA that can cause disease. A microarray test like karyotyping examines all chromosomes at once, but can detect changes that are smaller than karyotyping or FISH.

❖ 5- Gene expression profile: Gene expression profile examines whether genes are switched off in cells. Gene expression is the process of producing specific proteins from the information contained in genes. Different tissues express different genes based on their role in the body. The gene information is used to make a template for making RNA, and then the RNA is subjected to certain changes to create the protein needed by the cell. Genetics or genomics includes the analysis of genetic data and information, especially the genome of organisms. Genome is the entire DNA sequence in the cells of an organism, which acts as genetic material and causes hereditary traits to appear. By transferring hereditary material from one generation to another, hereditary traits are transferred from one generation to the next. In organisms that reproduce sexually, genes are passed to the baby through the male gamete and the female gamete. In short, it should be said that genomics includes the sequencing and analysis of genes and their transcripts in an organism.

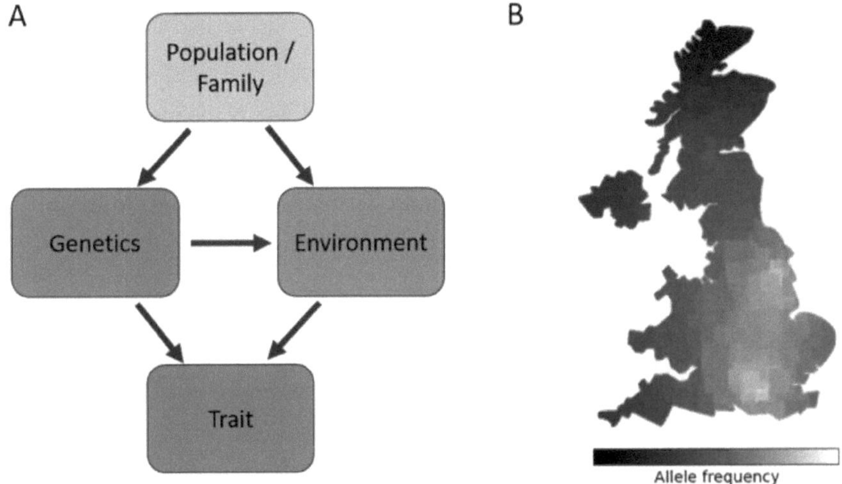

Figure 13. Open problems in human trait genetics

Genomics is the new face of genetics

One of the well-known scientific branches in the field of biology is genetics, which is actually the science of studying inheritance or transferring traits from one generation to another. Genes carry the necessary instructions to make proteins, which in turn determine the activities of the cell and different actions of the body, and in this way, they play a role in the occurrence of various traits. Recently, scientists have studied these genetic instructions in the form of a new field of science called genomics.

In fact, genomics is a new word that studies all the genes in the body of an organism and the interaction of these genes with each other and with the surrounding environment. In other words, genomics studies the sequence, structure and function of the genome. The focus of this new scientific branch is on the study and interpretation of genetic information or the organism's genome. This information includes the actions of each of the genes alone, the way of regulating their activity and how these genes are influenced by other genes and their surrounding environment.

Genomics is revolutionizing our understanding of living organisms from the molecular level to the cell, whole organism, and finally at the population level, advancing our understanding of evolution and the relationships between species. The set of activities of scientists in the field of genomics is carried out by using the new generation of scientific tools that help them determine the synonym or sequence of genes, the messages of these genes and their protein products, and finally the interpretation of the obtained information.

One of the stages of genomic investigations is the use of fast methods for gene sequencing, which is now done in most advanced laboratories with the help of robots and computers. The next step involves applying the information. A typical genome contains millions of pieces of genetic code. Researchers are currently using a computer kit and mathematical methods, collectively known as bioinformatics, to interpret, manipulate and analyze this information.

A global computer network called GRID is taking shape to allow scientists to access shared information and exchange and manipulate this genetic information a thousand times faster than was possible using the Internet. Other important steps of genomics include the preparation of genetic snapshots. Because at a certain time not all genes of an organism are active and it is possible to track the function of genes while they are active. Scientists need to make pictures of the function of genes during a certain process in progress in order to identify that process well.

One of the important points of laboratory investigations in the field of genomics is the use of model species. Individual genes and their location along chromosomes may be very similar in different species. Therefore, genomic studies in a number of model species provide information that can be used for other species as well.

For example, the results obtained from the study of fruit flies or yeast are also applicable to humans. If scientists find out exactly how the body reacts to tissue transplants, they will succeed in improving the transplant and cell repair systems, and finally, knowing the factors that determine the amount and type of chemicals made in a cell, will lead to better and new industrial biotechnology processes. will make it possible All these successes and advances are made in the shadow of benefiting from the new knowledge of genomics, and the molecular techniques used in genomics provide the possibility of studying biological systems with very high precision and sensitivity that could not be achieved before.

What is the difference between genetics and genomics?

Genetics is a term that refers to the study of genes and their role in heredity, and in other words, how some traits or conditions are passed from one generation to another. Genetics includes the scientific study of genes and their effects. Genes contain instructions for making proteins that direct cell activity and body functions. Examples of genetic or inherited disorders include cystic fibrosis, Huntington's disease, and phenylketonuria.

Genomics is a newer term that describes the study of all the genes of an individual, including the interaction of those genes with each other and with the surrounding environment. Genomics involves the scientific study of complex diseases such as heart disease, asthma, diabetes and cancer. Because these diseases are usually caused by a combination of genetic and environmental factors rather than just genes. Genomics offers new possibilities for treatment and treatment of some complex diseases as well as new diagnostic methods.

What is the importance of genetics and genomics for our health?

Both genetics and genomics play a role in our health and disease. Genetics helps people learn about how diseases like sickle cell anemia and cystic fibrosis are inherited, what screening and testing options are available, and, in some genetic conditions, available treatments. Genomics helps researchers understand why some people get sick and others respond differently to certain infections, environmental factors, and lifestyle behaviors.

For example, there are some people who exercise all their lives, eat a healthy diet, have regular medical check-ups, and die of a heart attack at the age of 40. There are also people who smoke, never exercise, eat junk food and live to be 100 years old. In fact, genomics can be the key to understanding these differences.

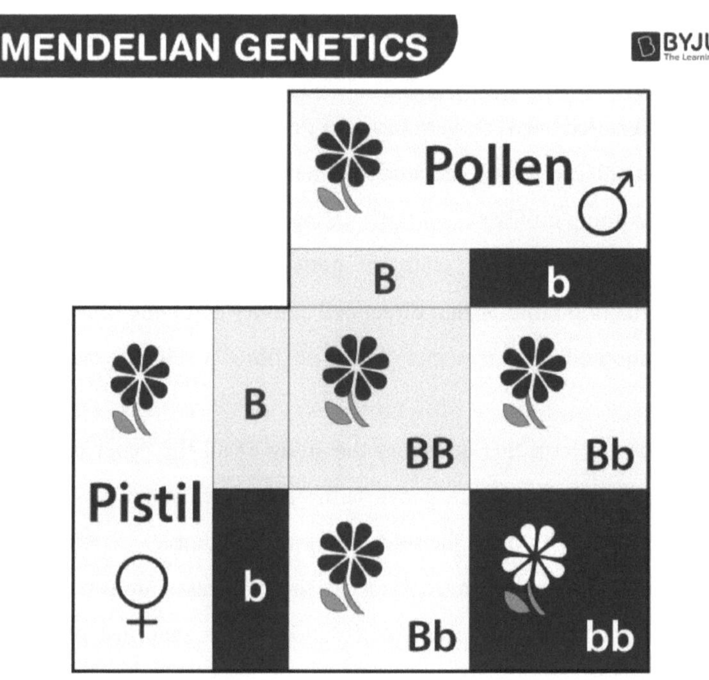

Figure 14. Mendelian Genetics Explore Mendel's Laws Of Inheritance

Apart from events, genetic factors are involved in 9 out of 10 leading causes of death in the United States. All humans are 99.9% identical in genetic structure. The difference in the remaining 0.1 percent has important clues about the causes of diseases. Gaining a better understanding of the interactions between genes and the environment using genomics will help researchers find better ways to improve health and prevent disease, such as modifying diet and exercise programs to prevent or delay type 2 diabetes. In people with a genetic predisposition to this disease.

Why is genetics and genomics important for family health?

Greater understanding of diseases caused by one gene using genetics and complex diseases caused by several genes and environmental factors using genomics can lead to faster diagnoses, interventions and targeted treatments. A person's health is influenced by family history and common environmental factors. This makes family history an important and personalized tool that can help identify many disease-causing factors that also have a genetic component. Family history can be the cornerstone of research on genetic and genomic conditions in a family, and the development of individual approaches to disease prevention, intervention and treatment.

New genetic and genomic techniques and technologies

1- Protozoology or proteomics (knowledge of examining the structure and function of proteins): the suffix -ome comes from the Greek language meaning all or complete. It was originally used in genome, which refers to all the genes of a person or other organism. Due to the success of large-scale biology projects such as the sequencing of the human genome, the suffix -ome is now used in other research fields as well. Proteomics is one such example. The DNA sequence of genes contains instructions or codes for making proteins. This DNA is transcribed into a related molecule called RNA and then translated into protein. Proteomics is therefore a large-scale, similar analysis of all proteins present in an organism, tissue type, or cell. Proteomics can be used to reveal specific and abnormal proteins that lead to diseases such as certain types of cancer.

2- Pharmacogenetics (pharmacology) and pharmacogenomics: the terms pharmacogenetics and pharmacogenomics are often used interchangeably to describe the intersection of the two scientific fields of pharmacology (the study of drugs) and genetic variation in determining a person's response to certain drugs. Pharmacogenetics is the field of study that deals with the variation in response to drugs due to variation in individual genes. Pharmacogenetics considers a person's genetic information about specific drug receptors and how drugs are transported and metabolized by the body.

The goal of pharmacogenetics is to create an individual drug therapy that allows the selection and best dose of the drug.

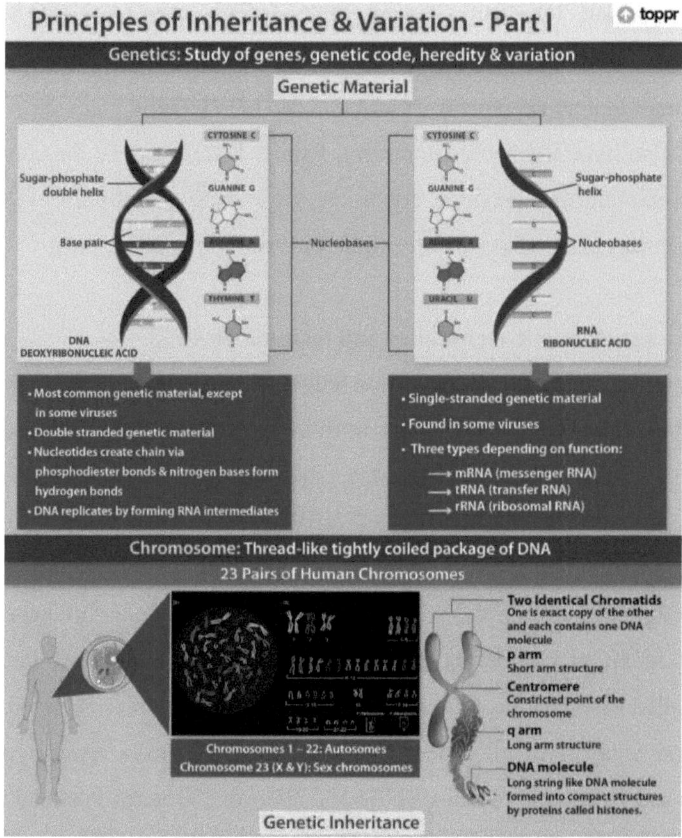

Figure 15. Genetics - DNA, RNA, Chromosome, Definition, and Videos

An example of this scientific field is the breast cancer drug Trastuzumab. This treatment only works for women whose tumors have a certain genetic profile that causes them to overproduce a protein called HER2. Pharmacogenomics is similar to pharmacogenetics, except that it usually involves looking for variations in several genes that are associated with variation in drug response. As pharmacogenomics is one of the large-scale omic technologies, it can examine the whole genome instead of individual genes. Pharmacogenomic studies may also examine genetic variation among large groups of people to see how different drugs may affect different racial or ethnic groups. Pharmacogenetic and pharmacogenomic studies lead to the development of drugs that can be tailored to specific individuals and adapted to each individual's specific genetic makeup. Although a person's environment, diet, age, lifestyle, and health status can also affect how that person's body responds to drugs, understanding a person's genetic makeup is key to creating personalized drugs that work better and have fewer side effects than conventional drugs. There are one-size-fits-all medications that are common today.

Treatment with stem cells: stem cells have two important features.
First: Stem cells are non-specialized cells that can transform into different body cells.
Second: that stem cells can remain in their unspecialized state and create copies of themselves.
Embryonic stem cells are obtained from the embryo in the early stages of development. Adult stem cells come from more fully developed tissues, such as cord blood in infants, circulating blood, bone marrow, or skin.
Today, medical researchers use stem cells to repair or replace damaged body tissues. Embryonic stem cells have the ability to transform from a blastocyst into any type of tissue found in an adult human. Mature stem cells are more limited in their potential. Stem cells have been used in experiments to form bone marrow, heart, blood vessel and muscle cells. Since the 1990s, cord blood stem cells have been used to treat heart problems and other physical problems in children with rare metabolic conditions, or to treat children with certain anemias and leukemias. For example, one of the treatment options for childhood acute lymphoblastic leukemia is stem cell transplantation.
There has been much debate about the use of embryonic stem cells, especially the creation of human embryos for use in experiments. In 1995, the US Congress passed a ban on government funding for research using human embryos. However, these limitations have not stopped researchers in the United States and elsewhere from using private funding to create and conduct research with embryonic cell lines. Such research

embryos are usually embryos created from eggs fertilized in vitro, such as in an in vitro fertilization clinic, and then donated for research purposes with the informed consent of the donors.

Cloning: Cloning can be about genes, cells or whole organisms. An allogeneic cell refers to any genetically identical cell in a population that descends from a single, common ancestor. For example, when a single bacterial cell copies its DNA and divides thousands of times, all the cells that are formed will contain the same DNA and be homologues of a common bacterial ancestor cell. Gene homology involves manipulations to create multiple identical copies of a single gene from a common ancestor. To homogenize an organism means to make an identical genetic copy of all the cells, tissues and organs that make up an organism. There are two main types of assimilation that may involve humans or other animals. One is therapeutic assimilation and the other is reproductive assimilation.

Allogeneic therapy involves growing cells or tissues that have been cloned from an individual, such as new liver tissue for a patient with liver disease. Such attempts at homogenization usually involve the use of stem cells. The nucleus is taken from a patient's body cell, for example, from a liver cell, and is placed in an egg whose nucleus has been removed.

This process eventually produces a blastocyst whose stem cells can be used to create new tissue that is genetically identical to the patient's tissue. Homologous reproduction is the process used to produce a complete animal that has the same nuclear DNA as the current or previous animal. The first homogenized animals were frogs. Dolly, a famous sheep, is another example of reproductive assimilation. However, the success rate of animal homogenization has been very low. In 2005, South Korean researchers claimed to have generated a human embryonic stem cell line by cloning genetic material from patients, but this data was later reported to have been falsified.

What is the application of data science in the field of genomics?

By delving deeper into the genome and analyzing and interpreting the collected genomic data, it will help to better understand human health and disease, but in the meantime, questions about privacy and ethics will also be raised.

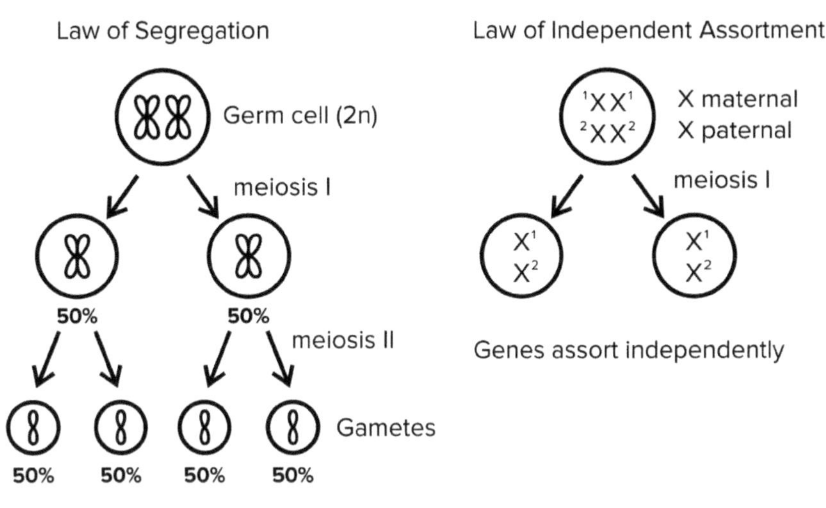

Figure 16. Genetics and Evolution for the MCAT:

Genomic data science is a field of scientific study that enables researchers to use powerful computational and statistical methods to decipher functional information hidden in DNA sequences.

Estimates predict that genomics research will generate between 2 and 40 exabytes of data in the next decade.

Our ability to sequence DNA is far greater than our ability to decipher the information contained within it. Therefore, genomic data science will be a dynamic research field for the coming years. Genomic data science components also carry a set of ethical responsibilities. Because each person's sequence data is also related to the privacy and identity issues of that person. With the rapid growth of biomedical research projects, the amount of genomic data generated is also increasing, so that currently approximately 2 to 40 billion gigabytes of data are generated each year. Researchers are trying to extract valuable information from such large and complex data sets in order to better understand human health and disease.

What is genomic data science?

Genomic data science is a field of study that enables researchers to use powerful computational and statistical methods to decipher functional information hidden in DNA sequences. These data science tools, used in the field of genomic medicine, help researchers and clinicians discover how differences in DNA affect human health and disease. Genomic data science emerged as a research field in the 1990s to bring together two laboratory activities:

1- Experiment: Generating genomic information from studying the genome of living organisms.

2- Data analysis: using statistical and computational tools to analyze and visualize genomic data, which includes processing and storing data and using algorithms and software to make predictions based on available genomic data.

Both activities help researchers to extract relevant information from large amounts of genomic dat

Why does genomics produce a lot of data?

Human genomics came into being in the early 1980s, when the Human genome project successfully created the first human genome sequence. Each trillion cells in the human body contains a complete copy of the genome, our DNA map. Most cells actually have two versions of the genome that reflect about 2 billion letters of DNA. Researchers now produce more genomic data than before to understand how the genome affects human health and disease. This data is obtained from millions of people in different populations around the world. Information about a human genome sequence alone occupies 2GB. It is estimated that we need 5 exhaust space to store genomic sequence data generated worldwide by year. It is good to compare that the five exabit can store all the words that humans have said. Due to the considerable volume of complex data related to the human genome, genomic is now considered as a macro-data string.

How do scientists' study genomic data?

Researchers need specific computational and analytical tools to find and interpret the biological information hidden in each person's DNA as well as manage the large amount of data produced in genomic research projects. Researchers use specific software tools called Aligners to determine the location of single pieces of DNA sequence in each part of a reference genome sequence. Next, when called Variant Callers, they identify places where a specific human genome sequence is different from other human genome sequences.

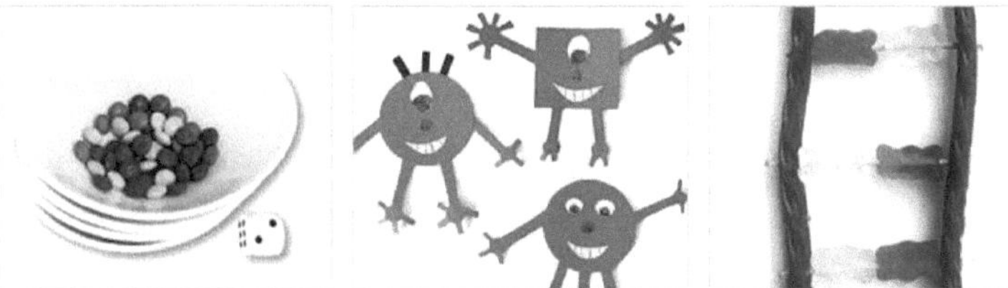

Figure 17. Teach About Genetics and Heredity with Free STEM Lessons & Activities

These genomic differences are of different sizes. This difference may be much larger as a small letter of a DNA, long letters such as insertions and deletions or chromosomal abnormalities. These genomic differences may have no danger to one's health, or can directly cause rare hereditary disorders, cancer or other more common diseases.

How do the researchers manage and store such a high volume of genomic data?
Computer and genomic technology experts manage and store genomic data using various computer systems and software. The increasing data analysis and coordination centers are part of these research networks and provide these services. Genomic data production requires a lot of financial support from institutions, such as the National Institute of Human Genome Research, which considers more than $ 5 million annually to support various genomic data efforts.

The produced data is often widely available to the scientific community to facilitate further data analysis. They organize and provide different types of information about the human genome, such as the location of different genes and species in DNA. Many private and commercial cloud platforms work in collaboration with government and public institutions such as the National Health Institute (NIH) through a group called Strides. These projects provide storage and computing infrastructure and security and privacy needed for genomic data.

What are the ethical, legal and social consequences for sharing genomic data?
Genomic research also has a set of ethical responsibilities. Because information about a person's genome sequence is related to complex issues related to privacy and identity.

1- **Consciousness:** Researchers usually receive satisfaction from people whose genomes have been sequenced, but they must provide clear information on how to use and share genome sequence data in the process of satisfaction.

2- **Privacy:** Powerful computational tools can obtain the sequence of identified genomes and, under special circumstances, connect them to the person whose DNA has been sequenced. Inspectors can use such tools for useful purposes, such as identifying criminals that have left DNA on the crime scene, but the social benefits of using genomic data should be greater than possible.

3- **Artificial Intelligence (AI):** Artificial intelligence tools are increasingly helping researchers processed a large number of genome sequence data to discover hidden patterns in DNA. This field of genomic data science requires extensive ethical research to examine the unique differences between current methods in genomic data science (which rely on human intelligence to interpret results) and newer methods of artificial intelligence. Although artificial intelligence methods provide very promising benefits, they conclude in completely different ways to humans, and therefore must be carefully monitored. With all these considerations, scientists and genomic researchers must learn about the consequences of their studies and closely collaborate with ethics researchers.

How do researchers share human genomic data?
Researchers are expected to share human genomic data based on participants' satisfaction. Genomic data is usually shared through data sources with a scientific community that can be accessed in three ways.

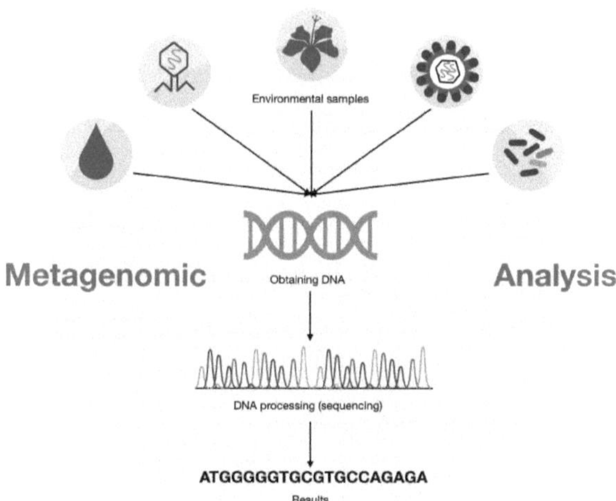

Figure 18. What is Genetics?

Types of access to genomic data

❖ **Free access or unlimited access:** which is the most extensive form of sharing. Data are publicly available to any research purpose.

❖ **Registered Access:** Located between open access and controlled access. In this case, the researchers can have data available for any purpose, provided they record their information and their work with data may need to be monitored.

❖ **Controlled Access:** In this case, data sharing requires that researchers describe the purpose of their research so that a specific access committee can evaluate the integration of the research with the participants' satisfaction. The researcher can only access data after receiving the committee's approval.

What are the new and emerging topics in the field of genomic data science?

The human genome contains many types of genomes. Health care systems and researchers are developing tools that identify these DNA differences and associate them with related medical information such as the risk of illness or a symptom for a particular drug. Researchers also use artificial intelligence systems to interpret genomic data for clinical purposes, such as diagnosing diseases in the early stages or predicting the risk of various diseases. In the past decade, cloud computing has been necessary for storing and analyzing genomic data. Cloud computing reduces the need to repeat large data set and increase security and allow researchers to access genomic data. Data scientists are creating tools to make data upload easier and guarantee privacy.

Five basic nutritional genomic principles

❖ Diet can be an important risk factor for different diseases in some people under certain conditions.

❖ Common chemicals in the diet change gene expression or genetic structure.

❖ The effect of diet on health depends on one's genetic composition.

❖ Some genes or types that may be involved in chronic diseases are adjusted using a proper diet.

❖ Diet-based diet-based interventions can be used to prepare an individual diet program focusing on health optimization as well as preventing or reducing chronic diseases.

The relationship between genetics and personal nutrition

Since personalized nutrition is new territory in relation to genetics, it is understandable that there is still much to learn in the scientific world. So don't worry about the details. Therefore, a few simple tips can be applied based on what has already been specified.

Properties of food sources and the importance of nutrition in genetic health

Nutrients prevent DNA damage (mutations). The following are important nutrients for preventing mutations that can lead to major diseases such as cancer or heart disease:

✓ Carotenoids such as: carrots, squash, yellow and red peppers, tomatoes and green leafy vegetables.

✓ Vitamin E such as: avocado, seeds and nuts.

Foods that facilitate DNA synthesis: There are foods that are important for the growth of hair cells, skin, nails, etc., and the growth of the fetus during pregnancy, and include folic acid, vitamin B12, zinc, and magnesium.

Foods that repair DNA: They are very important nutrients for repairing DNA mutation in our body and include vitamin B3 or niacin and folic acid.

It has been noted that different types of food provide beneficial properties for genetic health. It should also be noted that the group of foods consists not only of nutrients, but also of antioxidants, polyphenols, biologically active molecules, etc.

The relationship between intelligence, brain structure and genes

During human evolution, our brains have developed a lot. One of the regions that has developed over the last few million years is the cerebral cortex. This area processes sensory information and leads to movement, and is responsible for our high-level functions such as language processing and problem solving. Scientists focus on the structure of the cerebral cortex and discuss the reasons for its evolution throughout our lives and our evolution as a species to understand where heredity interacts with our intelligence. A new study of hundreds of developing brains has shown that there is a combination in certain areas of the cerebral cortex that develops from childhood to adulthood and is enhanced during adulthood and is linked to heredity.

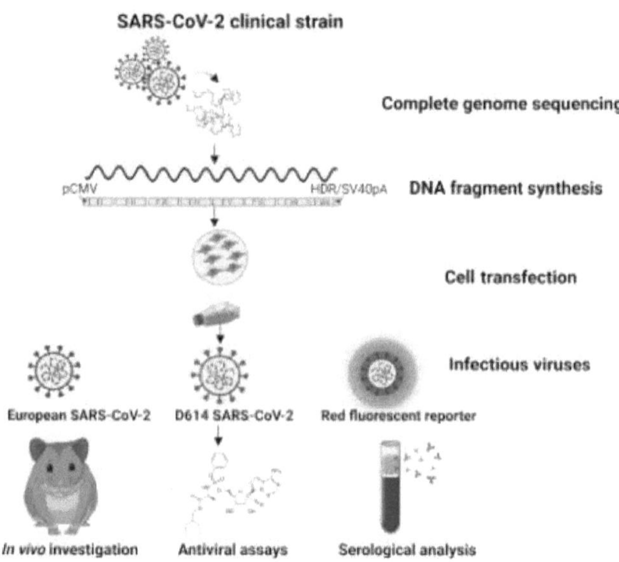

Figure 19. A simple reverse genetics method to generate recombinant coronaviruses

The scientists also found heritable relationships between IQ test scores and surface area in intelligence-related regions. Surface area of the brain shows the interaction between brain genes, intelligence and evolution.

An analysis of the brains of 600 children shows a connection between brain surface and heritability in brain regions important for cognition. During human evolution, our brains have become very large. One of these important areas that is highly developed is the cerebral cortex. The researchers also found a genetic link between IQ test scores and the surface area associated with intelligence, and this was published in the journal Neuroscience. "I think this is a big deal," said neuroscientist Rachel Brower at the University of Utrecht in the Netherlands. The authors of the study identified areas of the brain where variables are largely determined by genes, by examining neural connections and neurodevelopmental development. This is an attempt to relate heredity to the broader meaning of heredity.

New studies, new light on intelligence

Robert Lirk showed that most of the child's intelligence is based on the X chromosome and women have two X chromosomes. So, it is more likely that they carry genes related to intelligence. Carrying the intelligence gene does not mean that women have bigger and smarter brains. Based on scientific studies, it has been proven that the average brain of women is smaller than that of men. Being a superior gene carrier means that this gene can be passed on to the next generations, but it does not necessarily perform its function in the carrier's own body. In the previous parts, we explained that there are many genes that are activated in certain conditions. So, being a gene carrier does not mean the function of that gene in the body of the carrier. Recently, researchers from the University of Ulm in Germany investigated the genes responsible for brain degeneration and found that a large number of these genes, which are related to cognitive power, are located on the X chromosomes.

A remarkable result was obtained from a large analysis in Glasgow, Scotland. In this study, 12,686 young people between the ages of 14 and 22 were examined, and the researchers considered several factors, including facial color, the role of education in economic and social development, and economic status.

The researchers found that the most important determinant of average intelligence is the mother's intelligence, and they found that the average intelligence of young people is fifteen degrees different from their mother's intelligence. From the side of genes, we can see other studies that show that the mother plays an important role in the child's intellectual development through physical and emotional connection. In fact, studies show that safe communication between mother and child is significantly related to intelligence.

Researchers from the University of Minnesota found that children who developed strong relationships between themselves and their mothers were better able to learn complex puzzles, and these children were more stable and less likely to fail in solving problems. Because this strong connection gave children the necessary security to explore the world and confidence in solving problems, without losing their personality. In addition, mothers are interested in giving their children the highest support for solving problems, and this helps to increase their abilities. Researchers at the University of Washington have clarified the importance of emotional communication for brain development and discovered for the first time that communication with mother and mother's love is important for the development of some brain components. Scientists analyzed the way a mother communicates with her children for seven years and found that when the mother is emotionally supportive of the child and fulfills the child's intellectual and emotional needs in a sufficient amount, the hippocampus in children is ten percent larger than in children who do not. It is that they have been emotionally distant from their mother, and the hippocampus of the brain is related to memory and the ability to respond to emotional pressures.

This does not mean that we reduce the importance of the relationship with the father, but the reason for it is the social structure that causes some forms of growth and development in both sexes. This role difference between the two sexes is always present and it is usually the mother who spends most of her time with the child.

Can we talk about hereditary intelligence?

In fact, most measurements show that hereditary intelligence is between 40 and 60%, and this means that the remaining ratio is based on many factors, including the living environment, motivation, and personality traits. Intelligence is the power to solve problems, and surprisingly, the limbic system It plays an important role in solving problems, even if it is a simple physics or math problem. Because the brain acts like a single organ and thus intelligence has a deep connection with the power of rational thinking and is affected by the speed of thinking and emotions.

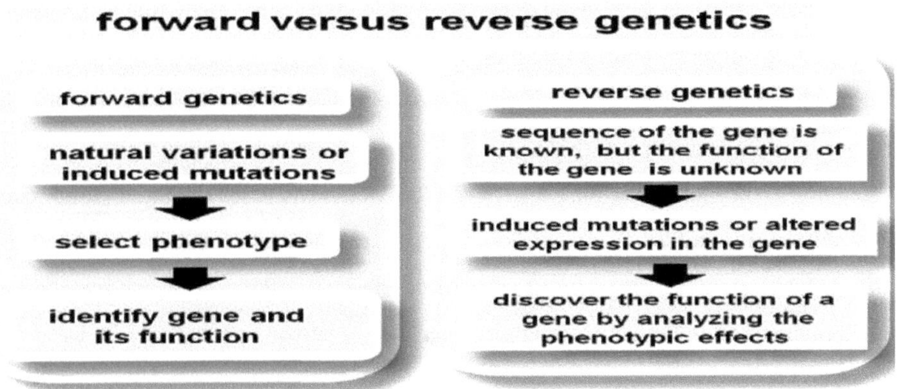

Figure 20. The difference between forward and reverse genetic techniques

In addition, we must not forget that even if a child's IQ is high, it is necessary to stimulate that intelligence throughout life. Because if intelligence is not stimulated with new stimuli, it will gradually decline and despite the effects of genes, it is appropriate to encourage fathers to contribute to the upbringing of children, especially from the emotional aspect.

The effect of genetics on obesity and overweight

Changes in the BNDF gene make people more inclined to eat high-fat foods and in large portions. In addition, these people are prone to obesity again after following a slimming diet. Therefore, they should continue their slimming diets and exercise in the long term so as not to gain weight again. Other tests that are recommended for obese people include:

- ✓ Genetic panel of susceptibility to diabetes.
- ✓ Genetic panel of amnesia and mental disorders.
- ✓ Appetite genetic panel.

The effect of genetics on weight fitness

Fat metabolism in the body is related to genetics. In fact, there is no direct relationship between diet and body weight. This means that some people consume a lot of food, but their weight does not increase compared to the food they consume, while some people gain a lot of weight by eating little food.

This difference is due to the effect of genetics on weight ratio. There is no doubt that both diet and physical activity play an important role in determining our weight, but according to recent studies, the cause of 40-70% of obesity cases is genetic. It has even been determined that the response of obese people to slimming diets with various sports also differs from each other. In other words, genes affect the absorption, metabolism and storage of fat in the body of people. Therefore, a person may become fat by eating a certain food.

What is the importance of genetic testing in the treatment of obesity?

By conducting special tests on each person's DNA, it is possible to find out if he carries certain genes that make him prone to overweight and obesity or not. Also, if you follow what kind of diet and which group of sports can you overcome obesity or overweight problems? A person will find out to what extent his obesity has a genetic background, and if obesity has genetic roots, the doctor can choose the best treatment method by finding out which of the person's genes are involved.

The diet is different for each gene. When a person is not aware of his genetic obesity, he may choose a diet that not only does not cause weight loss, but also aggravates the person's obesity. A person will find out whether physical activity and exercise are effective in losing weight or not? and which exercise should be done for his fitness? does the doctor easily determine whether drug treatment is useful for a person or not? The genes studied in the special test for the study of genes related to weight proportionality of 6 genes related to obesity are studied.

What is molecular genetic testing?

According to studies, changes in the FABP2 gene cause abdominal fat and resting metabolism. These people should avoid consuming saturated fatty acids and use more unsaturated fatty acids, especially omega3. In addition, the consumption of complex carbohydrates found in vegetables, bread and whole grains will also help in the metabolism of fats and increase insulin sensitivity.

Autosomal dominant inheritance pattern

The autosomal dominant trait has two specific characteristics. First, the one that is transmitted through asexual chromosomes, and the other one that manifests itself in the heterozygous state. In this case, if one of the parents has a dominant trait or disease, all his children have a 50% chance of inheriting that trait or disease. Examples of these diseases are Marfan, Huntington, muscular dystrophy.

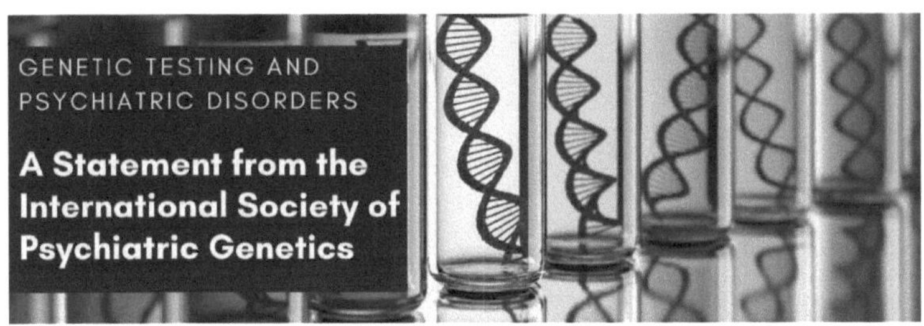

Figure 21. Genetic Testing Statement

These diseases have variable severity. In other words, clinical symptoms in different people can be different from one person to another. For example, in polycystic kidney disease, during which the kidney has multiple cysts. A person may show symptoms of the disease in early adulthood. However, another person can be without symptoms until the end of old age. The interesting thing about these diseases is that a person can look completely normal without any symptoms even though he is heterozygous. In this case, which is called reduced penetrance, during the passing of generations, the modifying effects of other genes as well as the interaction of genes with the environment can prevent the occurrence of symptoms.

For example, in people who have a mutated gene predisposing to breast cancer, the probability of cancer is 80%. In other words, due to the presence of other genes, the probability of the mutation of this gene has decreased by 20%. Another interesting point is that in some people with a dominant trait, parents can lack any dominant gene. In other words, a child with a dominant disease is born from parents who are completely healthy. In this case, following an error during gene transfer, a new mutation occurs. An example of this condition is achondroplasia, in which parents have a normal height, but their child has a form of dwarfism with short arms and legs. Regarding how to diagnose autosomal dominant disease with the help of genealogy, it should be kept in mind that sex chromosomes have no role in this disease.

Three Major Areas of Genetics		
Classical Genetics (Transmission)	Molecular Genetics	Evolutionary Genetics
Mendel's Principles	Genom	Quantitative Genetics
Meiosis + mitosis	DNA structure	Population Genetics
Sex determination	Chemistry of DNA	Evolution
Sex linkage	Transcription	Speciation
Chromosomal mapping	Translation	
Cytogenetics	Control of gene expression	
	DNA cloning	

Figure 22. Areas of Genetics

As a result, transmission between generations is carried out by people of both sexes, and in addition, the possibility of infection is equal between men and women. Finally, it is seen in autosomal dominant diseases of conflict in several continuous generations.

Chapter III

Study of Genetics

Mutations have a specific purpose and program towards a superior survival tool or intelligence tool, and mutations are not always random. In the previous sections, articles were written about the role of natural selection in correcting mutations that are incompatible with the environment, but the existence of this repair process to correct errors It does not mean that mutations are unplanned. There is an internal program in genes and chromosomes that can increase or decrease the speed of evolution even under similar environmental conditions. Even in a period of time with changing conditions, it can keep the speed of evolution improving.

The Neo-Darwinism theory of evolution by natural selection of random mutations should be consigned to history! Electromagnetic exchanges and communications may play a role in activating and causing mutations in healthy genes. This old theory has been challenged by directional mutations. The traditional Neo-Darwinism theory of evolution is based on the natural selection of random mutations along with the bigoted belief that environmental influences cannot change and inherit nucleic acids in a programmed way.

This fanatical belief was invalidated in the early 1980s with the advent of genetics and genome research. Similarly, the randomness of mutation was doubted until 1970 and shows that cells subjected to non-lethal selection are constantly exposed to which directional and adaptive mutations in specific genes; In a way that makes cells capable of life and reproduction. Note that mutations that are compatible for cells to enable them to grow and reproduce are not the same for the whole organism and can lead to tumors or cancer in some organs.

Therefore, it is better to call them directional mutations. In fact, it has been suggested that cancers may involve directional mutations, prompting John Karin to investigate this phenomenon in bacteria at Harvard University in Boston, Massachusetts. One of the first tests that showed directional mutations was on a species of E. coli bacteria with a mutation in the lacZ gene, which incompletely terminates polypeptide production; Therefore, the form that is mutated for lactose cannot use lactose only when lactose is present in the medium and not when lactose is not present in the medium. When there is no lactose, the bacteria gradually move towards repair mutations to make it possible to use lactose.

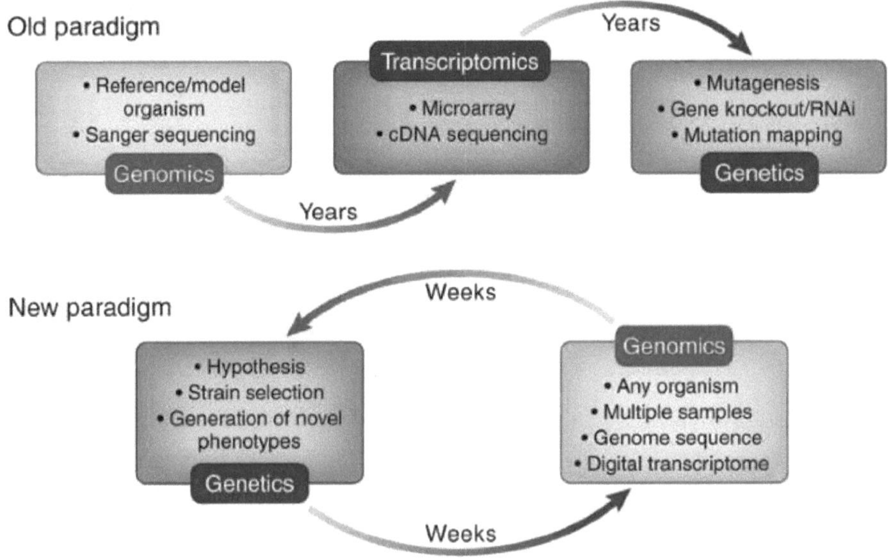

Figure 23. Fast forward genetics

Even more remarkable: A species in which the lacZ gene has been completely deleted can mutate the dormant gene ebgA and the regulatory gene ebgA that inhibits this gene and encodes the enzyme that hydrolyzes lactose. During the growth of each of these point mutations occur with a frequency of less than 8 to 10 and none of them will allow the species lacking lacZ to use lactose. But gradually, during lactose deficiency, these mutations increase to make it possible to use little lactose.

Karins and his colleagues concluded: When we consider what mechanisms might underlie the mutation described in this paper, we see that molecular biology is moving beyond the simplistic and the naturalistic. Now almost everything is possible in special systems!! Information is transferred freely from RNA to DNA. Genomic instability can change under stress conditions, and if the stress is too high, it can be completely shut down, and there are examples where cells can undergo many transformations and differentiations in certain regions of their genome. The most important category of communication that has yet to be described is between proteins and their constituent mRNA molecules. If a cell discovers how to make that connection, it may be able to test some options and chances based on which mutations are accepted or rejected based on it. When this happens, reverse translation as described by Karins and the same mechanisms for directional mutations can be transferred from E. coli bacteria to humans as new research shows.

It means an intelligent and conscious leap that is created beyond the influence and natural selection in the beginning to adapt the living being to its living environment. The creation of predictable mutation points based on secondary basic loop structures in single-stranded DNA provides in all cases transcription of a single-stranded DNA that presents unpaired internal mutable bases, and the mutable bases are guanine and cytosine.

Why they are mutagenic depends on the base-loop secondary structures (SLSs) that capture the transcribed single-stranded DNA and the strands that pair together are separated to release the unpaired bases as a loop. And these are the unpaired bases guanine and cytosine that are more prone to cause mutations. The MFG computer algorithm was used to simulate the environmental conditions in response to increased transcription speeds.

During transcription, open sensitivity for mutation is dependent on the stability of secondary SLSs on single-stranded DNA and the rate at which it is separated.

The mfg program has a two-way relationship with the mfold program and merges single-stranded fragments of specified length and chain and all possible secondary structures that can be created from each of the intermingled fragments in order of their stability reports mfg reports the stability of the more stable secondary structure in which the mutagenic base is not separated, as well as the amount of overall folds in the unpaired case. The mutagenic index of each unpaired base is the product of two variables: Guanine and cytosine in P53 and is basically located in the single-stranded

DNA loop of SLSs, and this is confirmed by analyzing codon 175 in exon 5 and using endonuclease s1. This enzyme cuts RNA and single-stranded DNA.

Unpaired guanine and cytosine are mutable, and unpaired guanine is mutated to adenine and unpaired cytosine is mutated to thymine. Evidence for background instability of unpaired guanine and cytosine is shown by examples of silent mutations that do not alter the amino acid chain. In all cases, the mutable bases are placed in the loops of known secondary structures.

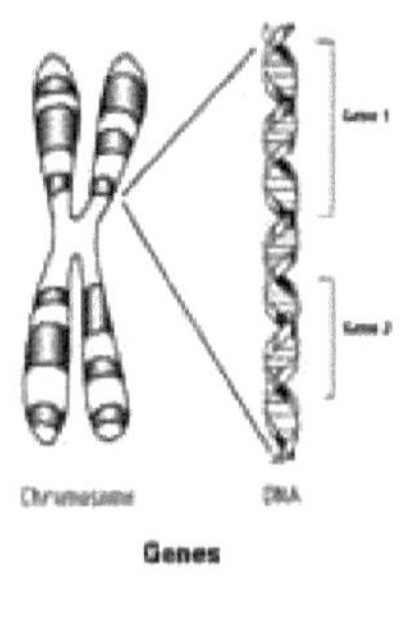

Figure 24. Basic genetics

Many somatic mutations (somatic hyper mutation) (SHM) are translated 10,000 times more in the precursors of B lymphocytes, and this, especially in phase 1 (somatic hyper mutation) (SHM), causes a million-fold increase in mutation frequency. An enzyme called deaminase Induced by activity that modifies RNA, it is involved in the mechanism of mutation in (somatic hyper mutation) (SHM) as well as in other systems. In hepatocellular carcinomas caused by toxin and P53 involvement, the availability of mutated and unpaired guanine. In single-stranded DNA, it changes the rate and frequency of mutations.

Environmental conditions at the transcription level show that most of the internal mutations are guanine to adenine, and the availability of guanine in single-stranded

DNA limits the rate of mutation frequency. The double effect of oxy radicals (reactive oxygen species that originates from incomplete oxidation) which increases the transcription about four times and increases the mutation of guanine to thymidine up to 85.8% is associated with the reduction of conversion and mutation of guanine to adenine. Therefore, oxygen radicals compete with rate-determining mutations.

Other evidence about non-random mutations

In humans, SHM and recombination of class and sample changes cause specific genetic changes in different regions of immunoglobulin genes in B lymphocytes in the production of antibody variants, point mutations in different regions and large deletions in switch regions. Both of them cause immune system disorder. Bcell stimulation, which induces CSR but not SHM, causes the accumulation of AID-dependent SHM-like point mutations in regions of mu alteration unrelated to CSR. These findings strongly suggest that AID (activation induced deaminase) itself or some individual molecules created by the action of RNA modifier on AID may mediate a general step of SHM and CSR and may be involved in breaking DNA. The human immune cells face the enemy, and before being affected by the enemy (or antigen) at a high speed, it creates certain genetic changes in its genes and makes an adaptive antibody to fight, and this antibody quickly enter the fight against the antigen.

This process is before the antigen can affect the genetic structure of the immune cells. This means that we are faced with an internal intelligence in the genetic structure that helps the protective cells of the body to prepare themselves to get rid of the invasion of antigens, and interestingly, the invading cell also undergoes intelligent genetic changes when faced with the host's defense system. It creates so that it can escape from the host's defense system. Another study suggests that double-stranded DNA breaks (DSBs) are responsible for mutational hotspots in stress-induced mutations in E. coli: The first produces mutations that occur most abundantly in the first 2,000 bases and logarithmically up to 60 It is reduced a thousand times.

The latter involves a weak mutational continuation that reaches up to one million bases from the double chain break. Critical points in the replication path move up and down independently. Rec D enzyme, which allows DSB-exonuclease activity, is required for strong regional mutations and long-distance hotspots, and shows that double-strand separation and gap-filling synthesis underlies hotspot mutations.

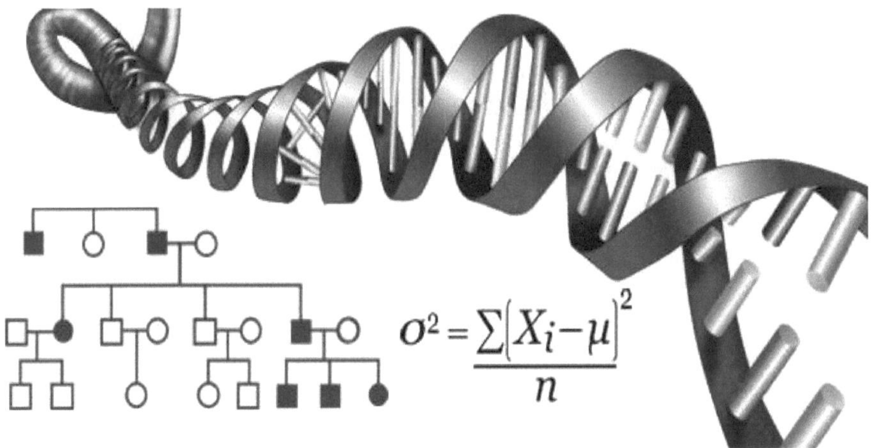

Figure 25. Statistical Genetics and Genetic Epidemiology

Sensitive points near DSB open the possibility that specific genomic regions can be targeted to cause mutations and can cause simultaneous evolution in genes and genetic groups. At the end of a study that connects population genetic techniques and breeding and compares up to 34 E. coli genomes, it was conducted by researchers at the European Institute of Bioinformatics (breeding is a branch of biology that studies the evolutionary relationship of different groups. organisms such as species or populations). The study showed that the rate of natural mutations; Whether it is beneficial or non-beneficial, it changes within 2,659 genes, and the hot and cold points of mutation extend over several kilo bases.

The changes are not random, the rate is lower in genes that are highly expressed and displayed, and in genes that have a stronger refining selection, and this shows that they are preferentially protected from mutations or by repair mechanisms.

These findings suggest that the mutation rate is evolutionarily regulated to reduce the risk of dangerous mutations. However, new knowledge of the factors that affect the rate of mutation, including repair along with transcription and the creation of position-dependent mutations. It does not explain the observation and indicates that other processes must exist.

More than 12,000 single nucleotide polymorphisms have been tested. Considering that transcription is mutagenic and causes mutations (based on the studies previously stated), a negative relationship between the manifestation and the rate of mutation is not expected, and this indicates that there are ways of repair along with transcription. But this process alone is not enough because the un transcribed chain also shows the relationship between manifestation and mutation rate, and molecular tests have reported that mutagenesis exists in the presence of transcription along with repair. Therefore, there must be other mechanisms that generally involve genes with high expression, but are not directly associated with the transcription machinery.

How does the cell know which gene is mutated? The findings show that there are many mechanisms for the cell to make direct mutations in specific genes and specific regions in these genes, but they do not provide any reason as to how the cell does this. I suggest electromagnetic messages are involved.

There are good reasons to assume that molecules communicate with each other through electromagnetic messages, and that molecules that communicate emit common frequencies; So they can attract each other through resonance. If this is the case, lactose, which is supplied in small amounts during starvation, sends strong electromagnetic messages to its normal metabolic enzyme B-GALACTOSIDASE and its gene LACZ, and this causes it to respond to transcription and attract the necessary magnetic machine. So that the gene can be transcribed and translated into an enzyme that breaks down lactose and thus restores normal metabolic flow.

A similar case exists in other stress conditions and stress recovery. The amplification of electromagnetic messages is very accurate and will have all the views in a directional manner; Especially if the cell and the organism are quantum compatible. This hypothesis can be tested and the messages can be shown with detectors (sensors) and sensitive analyzers. Mutations are highly non-random and directional. Several mechanisms are used to create mutations and are under the control of the cell or organism as a fabric in a different environmental context, and this causes reproducible mutations in certain genes. These results are contrary to the Neo-Darwinism view, in which evolution depends on the natural selection of random genetic mutations. In my opinion, the electromagnetic messages that are emitted by key molecules that can eliminate stress are directly related to activate the transcription and transcription of the required genes.

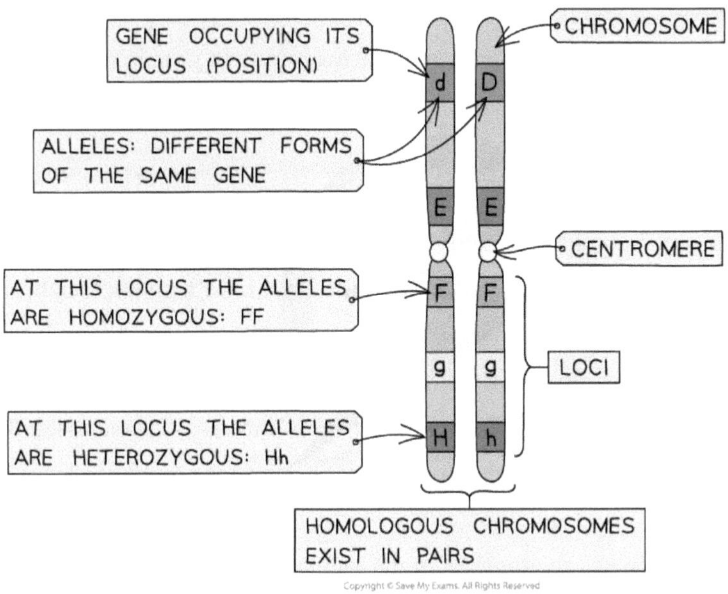

Figure 26. Key Terms in Genetics (16.2.1)

Seyyed Ahmad Al-Hassan says in the book "The Illusion of Atheism": Mutation is lawful and purposeful, and it is based on the internal law of the genetic map, and it is not completely blind or only based on blind causes! In the case of chromosomes, there is a law that determines the speed of mutation, and in a clearer sense, the genetic map is legal, and therefore it creates many mutations in a certain direction in a certain period of time; In such a way that it puts pressure on the path of evolution and causes it to accelerate and move at a high speed until it reaches a certain goal in a certain period of time of evolution or we can say new species or species, then the speed of the mutation jumps to a standstill or very fast. It comes back slowly and the evolution comes back to this slow speed along with it, because evolution is based on mutations and without evolutionary mutation, it is not possible to imagine, and maybe it is not a rare example of the Cambrian period or the Cambrian explosion.

Rather, it may be the evolution of the human brain in the last two million years, and the logical interpretation of the increase in the rate of mutation towards the increase in brain size in humans or Homo sapiens in the last two million years is that the mutation is lawful and purposeful and based on the internal law of the genetic map. And not completely blind or only based on blind causes such as errors in genetic copying and being broken by cosmic rays.

The role of genetics in cancer

The purpose of genetic testing is to identify specific hereditary changes (mutations) in a person's chromosomes and genes. Genetic mutations may have harmful, beneficial, ineffective, or uncertain effects on a person's health status. Deleterious mutations may increase a person's chance or risk of developing a certain disease, such as cancer. In total, inherited mutations are involved in about 5-10% of cancers. In some cases, the accumulation of cancer is seen in some families, but the cause is not the existence of hereditary mutations.

For example, the same living environment or the same way of life, such as smoking, may lead to the occurrence of similar cancers in family members.

However, the presence of some specific patterns such as the type of cancer, the presence of some non-cancerous diseases and the age of occurrence of each specific cancer may suggest the presence of hereditary cancer. Genetic mutations are known to cause hereditary cancers, and genetic tests can confirm whether the cancer is caused by a genetic mutation or not. In addition, conducting genetic testing in other family members who do not have obvious manifestations of the disease will determine whether they carry the same mutation that is known to be predisposed to cancer in their family or not. Hereditary genetic mutations can increase a person's risk of cancer through various mechanisms.

Does every person carrying a cancer-prone mutation necessarily get cancer?

Even if there is a mutation in a cancer-prone gene in the family, it does not necessarily mean that everyone who inherits this mutation will develop cancer. Various factors are effective in the outcome of a person with a mutation. An important factor is the inheritance pattern of hereditary cancer in the family.

In order to understand how cancer is inherited in the family, it is necessary to mention that each person has two copies of most genes and each copy is inherited from one of the parents. Most of the effective mutations in hereditary cancers are inherited with two patterns: Autosomal dominant and autosomal recessive. In autosomal dominant inheritance, the presence of one copy of the altered gene is enough to increase the probability of developing cancer in a person. In this case, one of the parents who transmitted the mutation may also show manifestations of the gene mutation. In autosomal recessive inheritance, only if a person inherits a copy of a defective gene from each parent, the risk of cancer will increase. Each parent has a defective and a healthy copy of the desired gene, and usually they are not at an increased risk of developing cancer.

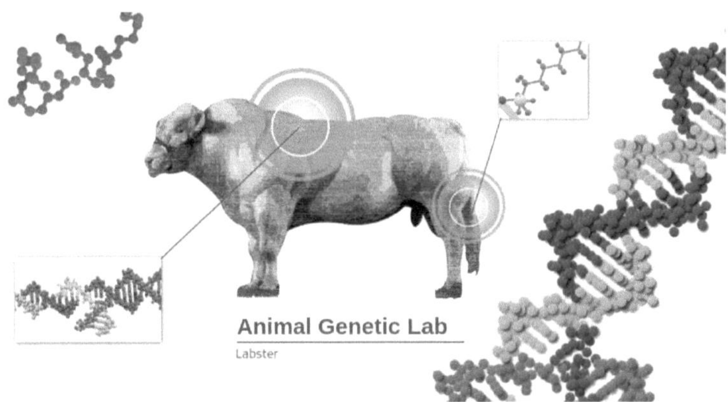

Figure 27. Animal Genetics

These parents are called carriers. Even when people have one autosomal dominant mutation in a cancer predisposing gene or two autosomal recessive mutations in a cancer predisposing gene, they may still not get cancer. Some mutations have incomplete penetrance, which means that the effects of the mutation can only be seen in some people. In addition, mutations may have different manifestations (Variable Expression). That is, the severity of symptoms may be different in different family members.

What genetic tests are available to determine cancer risk?

More than 50 hereditary cancers are known. Most of these cancers are caused by highly penetrant mutations that have autosomal dominant inheritance. Below are some examples of common hereditary cancers for which genetic testing is possible:

Hereditary breast and ovarian cancer

Genes: BRCA1 and BRCA2

Related cancers: Breast cancer in women, ovarian cancer and related cancers: Including prostate cancer, pancreas and breast cancer in men

Hereditary colon and rectal cancer

Genes: MSH2, MLH1, MSH6, PMS2, EPCAM and APC

Related cancers: Colon and rectal cancer, endometrial (womb) cancer, ovarian cancer, kidney cancer, pancreatic cancer, small intestine cancer, stomach cancer, liver and bile duct cancer, brain cancer, breast cancer and some skin lesions.

Genetic counseling

It is recommended that people consult a genetic specialist before deciding to do genetic tests. Genetic counseling helps people determine their cancer risk, benefits, and limitations of genetic testing for their specific condition. In some cases, the geneticist advises that it is not necessary to carry out a genetic test. Genetic counseling includes a complete review of individual and family medical history to determine the risk of cancer. During the counseling session, the following are also discussed:

> Is genetic testing appropriate? What specific tests may be used and how accurate is each test?

> What are the medical effects of a positive or negative test result?

> The possibility that the test result is not clear is raised, that is, the test result may not help to make medical decisions.

> What are the psychological benefits and risks of knowing the result of the genetic test?

> What is the risk of passing on the genetic mutation to the children?

Unlike many medical tests, genetic tests can reveal information not only about the person himself but also about his relatives. The presence of a harmful genetic mutation in a family member raises the possibility that other blood relatives may also carry that mutation. In some cases, some family members may want to know about their genetic status while others may have a different opinion. Counseling with a geneticist may help family members better understand the outcome of each of these choices.

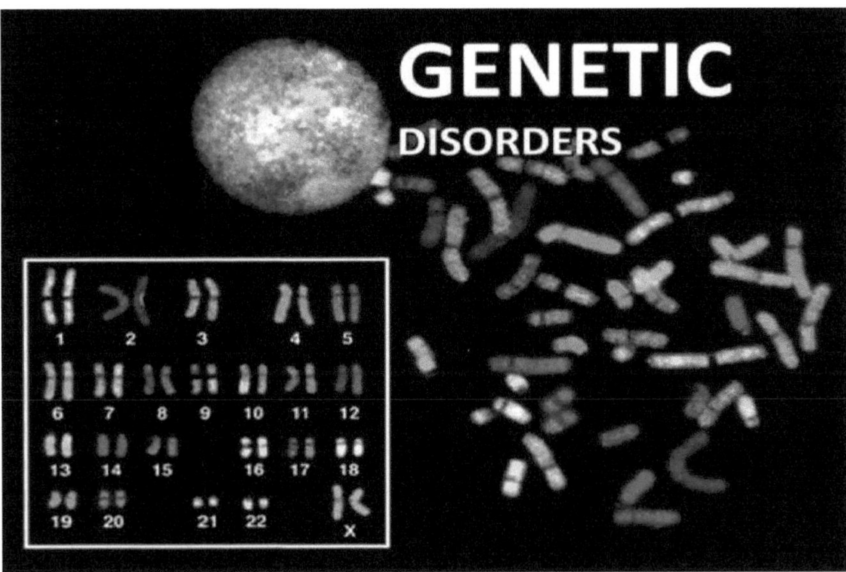

Figure 28. Pathology cptr5-genetics

Chapter IV

Normal cells and hyperplastic cells

Metastatic cells

At each stage, a specific gene (oncogene or anti-oncogene or repair gene) can mutate so that these cells become cancerous. If cancers are diagnosed in the first stages, they are completely curable, and if they are diagnosed in the second stages, they have a 70% chance of treatment, and if they are diagnosed in the third stages, they have a 30% chance of recovery, and if cancer is diagnosed, it is in the fourth stage, which has definitely spread to other tissues.

The chance of treatment and recovery is about 5% if it lasts for 5 years. These patients are treated in several ways. Surgery, chemotherapy, radiation therapy, immunotherapy and gene therapy, which is bone marrow transplantation. All these treatment methods have side effects on other healthy body tissues. Many environmental factors that produce cancer can be prevented, such as smoking, alcoholic beverages, polluted air, unhealthy diet, inactivity and infectious diseases, if aging and family genetics cannot be changed and prevented. Research in oncology today has helped us not only to better understand the function of cancer disease but also to provide the best treatment solution for these patients.

In the last three decades, researchers have reported a lot of information about genes and proteins and their role in the production of normal and cancer cells. One of their important discoveries was the role of mutated genes in the production of cancer cells. Environmental factors that because genetic mutations are being identified. With the help of different molecular methods, we are able to determine the expression strength of defective genes and proteins. Even finding new biomarkers that are an indicator of a type of cancer helps in early diagnosis and timely treatment of cancer disease. After determining the spatial forms of defective proteins, new anti-cancer drugs can be made that can target cancerous cells in order to prevent their production and growth into cancer cells.

Milestones in the history of cell theory

1665: Robert Hooke first described the cells he observed in cork (dead tissue).

1667: Van Leeuwenhoek observed and described bacteria and other microbes using a primitive microscope. At that time, many people believed that microbes were produced spontaneously.

1765: Spallanzani was the first to show that organisms do not arise spontaneously. He boiled a piece of meat with water and closed the lid of the container, the broth in the container remained clear. Proponents of spontaneity argued that the absence of air in a closed container prevented the growth of microbes in that container.

1838: Mathias Schleiden proposed after microscopic observations that plants are composed of units called cells.

1839: Theodor Schwann made a proposal similar to Schleiden's about animal tissues.

1858: Rudolf Virchow proposed a theory that became accepted as the cell theory: "Each animal is a collection of vital units, each of which has all the characteristics of a living being."

1864: Louis Pasteur repeated Spallanzani's experiment using a strong-necked glass (a tube with a long, narrow and winding neck) that allowed air to enter the broth, which discredited the theory of spontaneous generation.

Milestones in the history of genetics

460 BC: Hippocrates observed that traits and diseases have a hereditary component.

1859: Charles Darwin presented his theory about the evolution of organisms by means of natural selection, which has unified various organisms.

1860: The role of sperm and egg cells in reproduction was determined.

1865: Gregor Mendel identified the dominant and latent traits and also invented laws to understand heredity, which are known today as Mendelian laws.

1868: Eduard Hegel discovered that the sperm was a cell composed mostly of nuclear material and postulated with certainty that the nucleus was responsible for heredity.

1871: Frederic Miescher discovered nucleic acid, DNA, in the nucleus of cells that he got from a pus wound.

1875: Hertog observed the fertilization of animals and accepted as a principle of certainty that each cell nucleus is derived from another nucleus.

1879: Walter Fleming described the duplication of chromosomes in the nucleus.

1900: Carl Korns, along with Eric Chermack and Hugo Vries, each separately rediscovered Mendelian laws.

1903: Walter Sutton discovered that each gamete receives one of the two chromosomes from each pair of chromosomes present in a diploid cell. He accepted as a principle of certainty that genetic information is contained in chromosomes.

1908: Thomas Morgan researched Drosophila and proved that the gene is the unit of hereditary information and can be changed by mutation. Nobel Prize winner in 1933.

1909: Walter Johansen popularized the name gene for the hereditary unit.

1927: Hermann Müller and Louis Stadler separately showed that X-rays could induce mutations in Drosophila. Hermann Muller won the Nobel Prize in 1946.

1941: George Biddle and Edward Tatum proposed that each gene is responsible for the production of an enzyme by researching the mold Neurospora crassa. Nobel Prize winners in 1958.

1943: Luria and Delbork proved that the bacterium Escherichia coli can spontaneously become resistant to bacterial viruses. This discovery changed the face of genetic science and marked the beginning of the victory of Escherichia coli bacteria as the lifeblood of genetic research. Luria and Delbrook, Nobel Prize winners in 1969.

1944: Oswald Avery, Colin McLeod, and MacLean McCarthy, by researching the bacterium Pneumococcus pneumonia, settled the long-standing scientific debate that DNA is the material of heredity.

1945: Delbrook started the phage school (the study of viruses, parasites and microbes) in Cold Spring Harbor, USA, which had a tremendous impact on genetics and molecular biology. Delbrook won the Nobel Prize in 1969.

1949: Eric Chargoff discovered that the adenine content of the DNA molecule is equal to its thymine content and the guanine content is equal to its cytosine content, but the amount of A+T in the DNA molecule of different species of organisms is different.

1950: Maurice Wilkins and Rosalyn Franklin take the first X-ray pictures of DNA, showing that DNA has a regular structure.

1951: McLintock proved with corn research that some genes can move from one point to another in a chromosome. McLintock won the Nobel Prize in 1983.

1952: Hersky and Chips discovered that DNA is the genetic material of bacterial viruses. The number of those who were still in favor of the protein content of the genetic material was reduced. Hersky won the Nobel Prize in 1969.

1953: Francis Crick and James Watson interpreted Wilkins and Franklin's photographs of the DNA molecule and proposed a double helix structure for that molecule. These scientists proposed that this type of structure allows the DNA molecule to replicate in a very simple way. Francis Crick and James Watson, Nobel Prize winners in 1962.

1953: Luria, Yeoman, Bertani and Weigel discovered the phenomenon of restriction and modulation, which led to the discovery of restriction enzymes in molecular techniques. Luria won the Nobel Prize in 1969.

1956: Francis Crick proposed the central principle of molecular biology: Protein $\rightarrow$ mRNA $\rightarrow$ DNA. Francis Crick also proposed the existence of a "adapter" molecule that makes it possible to read mRNA during its translation into protein, which today is called tRNA. Francis Crick won the Nobel Prize in 1962.

1961: Urgel, Brenner and Crick, as a result of their study of bacterial viruses, determined that the genetic code is a triplet sequence.

1961: François Jacob and Jacques Monad proved that gene activity in E. coli should be regulated by external factors and proposed the first gene expression regulation model. Jacob and Monad, Nobel Prize winners in 1965.

1970: Mitzotani, Baltimore and Temin discovered by researching viruses that the central principle of Francis Crick's proposal should be modified. There is an enzyme called reverse transcription enzyme or reverse transcriptase that can synthesize a double-stranded DNA molecule from a single-stranded RNA molecule. Temin and Baltimore Nobel Prize winners in 1975.

1977: Roberts and Sharp discovered the existence of introns in eukaryotes. Nobel Prize winners in 1993.

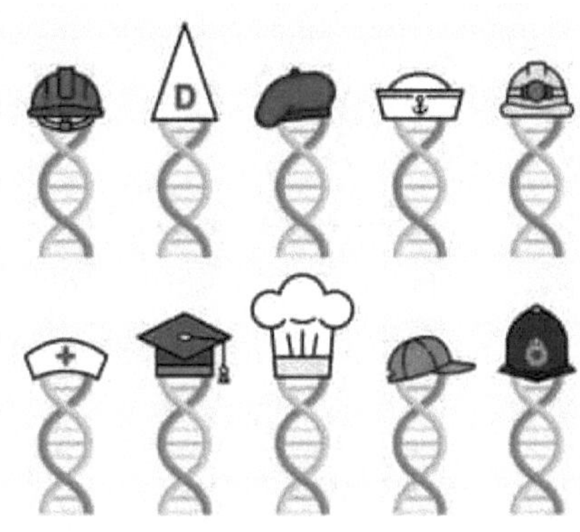

Figure 29. So, is it nature not nurture after all?

Milestones in Biochemical History Related to Genetic Science

1828: Wehler first synthesized urea, which is an organic molecule, in the laboratory. Urea is found in animal urine. This discovery showed that organic materials can be synthesized from inorganic materials. The end of vitalism research.

1857: Louis Pasteur first demonstrated the enzymatic reaction in a microscopic organism. During wine fermentation, glucose is converted into ethanol in the yeast cell.

1897: Buchner was the first to show the enzymatic reaction in a test tube; Glucose is converted into ethanol by the extract of yeast cells and in the absence of living cells. Nobel Prize winner in 1907.

1900: Fischer proposed that the amino acids of the protein molecule are connected by chemical bonds. Nobel Prize winner in 1902.

1926: George Sumner was the first to purify the urease enzyme that breaks down urea. Nobel Prize winner in 1946.

1949: Pauling proved that sickle cell anemia was caused by an abnormal hemoglobin molecule. Nobel Prize winner in 1954.

1949: Brecht and Casperson discovered that RNA is located in the cytoplasm of eukaryotic cells and is also the site of protein synthesis.

1953: Frederick Sanger determined the amino acid sequence of a type of protein called insulin for the first time. Today, Sanger sequencing is used in nucleotide sequence. Winner of the Nobel Prize in 1958.

1956: Korenberg proved that the DNA molecule could be duplicated in a test tube. Nobel Prize winner in 1959.

1957: Ingram showed that the hemoglobin of patients with sickle cell anemia differed by only one amino acid from the hemoglobin of healthy individuals. After the discovery of the genetic code, it became possible to observe that the change of just one nucleotide can make a person sick.

1956-58: Zemneck and Hoagland discovered the adapter molecule hypothesized by Francis Crick, now called transfer RNA.

1961: Three different laboratories isolated the mRNA molecule.

1965: Arber proved that the restriction phenomenon is caused by the presence of an enzyme that cuts DNA but not precisely. Nobel Prize winner in 1978.

1970: Smith first isolated the restriction enzyme that cuts the DNA molecule at a very specific nucleotide. Nobel Prize winner in 1978.

The beginning of the era of genetic engineering

1973: Cohen and Bayer synthesized the first recombinant DNA.

1977: Maxam and Gilbert and Sanger discovered two different methods for DNA sequencing. Maxam and Gilbert won the Nobel Prize in 1980. Frederick Sanger won the Nobel Prize in 1958 and 1980.

1983: Gary Mullis discovers the polymerase chain reaction (PCR) technique that converts a piece of DNA into millions of copies in a relatively short time. Nobel Prize winner in 1993.

1987: Smith made a gene mutate in a test dish and then reintroduced it back into a living cell. Nobel Prize winner in 1993. Milestones in the history of human genetics

1900: Karl Landsteiner presented the ABO blood group system to mankind. With this great discovery, blood transfusion became possible without risk and safe between humans. Nobel Prize winner in 1930.

1902: Garo studied one of the human diseases, Alkaptonuria. The patient excretes homogentic acid in his urine, which is seen in dark color near the air.

By studying the family trees of the patients' families, Garrow realized that the laws of inheritance that Mendel had discovered provided a reasonable explanation of this phenomenon, which corresponded to the mode of inheritance of latent traits. Garo was the first to suggest the relationship between a genetic defect and the absence of an enzyme.

Despite the fact that Garrow held an honorary chair of medicine at Oxford University, the value of his creative contribution to the science of human genetics remained unknown during his lifetime. Biologists did not pay much attention to the work of a doctor, and the medical world did not understand the importance of Garo's findings for medicine.

1911: Van Dungeren and Hirschfeld demonstrated the ABO mode of inheritance of the blood system, which is a striking example of the application of Mendelian inheritance to a human trait.

1911: Frederick Roos was the first discoverer of a virus that causes cancer in domestic animals or chickens, the "Roos Sarcoma" virus. Nobel Prize winner in 1966.

1956: Tejo and Luan proved that humans have a total of 46 chromosomes.

1959: Legion reported that Down syndrome may be caused by having three copies of chromosome 21 instead of the normal two.

1965: Harris and Afroosi developed methods for fusing mouse and human cells. With this work, it became possible to determine the location of many genes in special chromosomes. Since then, other methods have been developed, and today, more than 23,000 human genes that encode proteins with known functions have been mapped.

1980: Bishop and Varmus proved that viruses can induce some types of cancer in humans. Nobel Prize winners in 1989.

1981: Wirgler first isolated a gene from humans that causes cancer when mutated.

1990: Blaise, Culver, and French Anderson performed gene therapy for the first time at the National Institutes of Health in Bethesda, USA.

From two hundred thousand years ago, when the first human civilization appeared on earth, until now, mankind has always tried to understand the secrets of life due to his inner curiosity towards everything that was unclear to him, and today, the same techniques that the human hand has invented the way and method of thinking easier and faster, and everything that was once vague and dumb for humans, has been covered with practicality today.

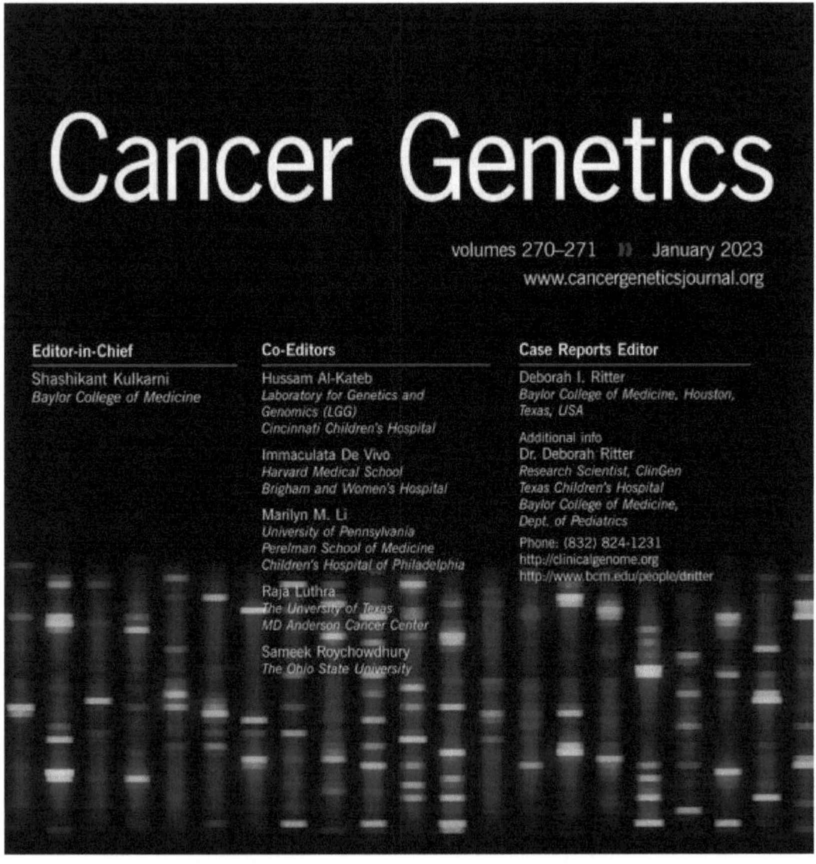

Figure 30. Home Page: Cancer Genetics

What is genetic testing?

Genetic testing is the laboratory analysis of the genetic material of the human body. This test involves chromosomes, deoxyribonucleic acid (DNA) or ribonucleic acid (RNA) to detect genetic material and/or identify genetic changes. Certain segments of DNA, called genes, act as templates for building (transcribing) RNA. Genetic changes are referred to as "mutations" (sometimes called "mutations") and can have different effects on the body. Although most genetic changes do not affect a person's health, they are sometimes associated with disease.

How is genetic testing done?

To perform a genetic test, some kind of body sample is required. This sample can be blood, urine, saliva, body tissues, bone marrow, hair, etc. The sample can be received in a tube, on a swab in a container or frozen. After that, in a specialized laboratory, the genetic material is isolated and removed from the sample. Some genetic disorders are linked to a single gene, and genetic testing naturally focuses on testing mutations in genes based on symptoms or a person's family history.

For example, cystic fibrosis has a well-defined set of symptoms, and testing for mutations in a single gene can usually identify the cause of these symptoms. However, there are many other genetic disorders that are not easily recognized. These are linked to several genes or large parts of the genome. The following sections provide an overview of genetic testing methods, ranging from identifying or examining a single gene to the entire genome.

Genetic testing methods

- PCR
- DNA sequence
- Cytogenetics (karyotype and FISH)
- Microarrays
- Gene expression profiling.

Gene expression profiling

Gene expression profiling examines whether or not genes are turned off in cells. Gene expression is the process of producing specific proteins from the information contained in genes. Different tissues express different genes based on their role in the body. Gene information is used to make a template for making RNA. The RNA is then subjected to specific changes to create the protein needed by the cell.

Genealogy or genomics (in French: génomique) includes the analysis of genetic data and information, especially the genome of organisms. Genome is the entire DNA sequence present in the cells of an organism, which acts as genetic material and causes the appearance of hereditary traits (phenotype).

By transferring hereditary material from one generation to another, hereditary traits are transferred from one generation to the next. In organisms that reproduce sexually, genes are transferred to the baby through the male sex cell (sperm) and the female sex cell (ovum). In short, it should be said that genomics includes the sequencing and analysis of genes and their transcripts in an organism.

Genomics is the new face of genetics

One of the well-known scientific branches in the field of biology is genetics, which is actually the science of studying inheritance or transferring traits from one generation to another. Genes carry the necessary instructions to make proteins, which in turn determine the activities of the cell and various actions of the body, and in this way, they play a role in the occurrence of various traits.

Recently, scientists have studied these genetic instructions in the form of a new field of science called genomics. In fact, genomics is a new word that studies all the genes in the body of an organism (genome) and the interaction of these genes with each other and with the surrounding environment.

In other words, genomics studies the sequence, structure and function of the genome. The focus of this new branch of science is on the study and interpretation of genetic information or the organism's genome. This information includes the actions of each gene alone, the way their activity is regulated, and how these genes are affected by other genes and their environment.

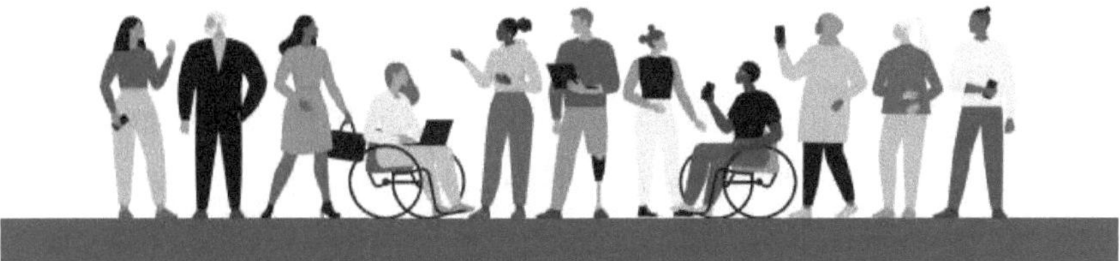

Figure 31. Genetic Risk

Genomics is revolutionizing our understanding of living organisms from the molecular level to the cell, the whole organism, and finally at the population level, advancing our understanding of evolution and the relationships between species. The activity of scientists in the field of genomics is carried out using the new generation of scientific tools that help them determine the synonyms or sequence of genes, the messages of these genes and their protein products, and finally the interpretation of the obtained information.

One of the stages of genomic investigations is the use of fast methods for gene sequencing, which is now done in most advanced laboratories with the help of robots and computers. The next step involves using information.

A typical genome contains millions of pieces of genetic code. Researchers are currently using a computer kit (laboratory package for a specific purpose) and mathematical methods collectively called bioinformatics to interpret, manipulate and analyze this information. A global computer network called GRID is being formed to allow scientists to access and manipulate shared genetic information a thousand times faster than was possible using the Internet. Other important steps of genomics include the preparation of genetic snapshots. Because at a certain time all the genes of an organism are not active and it is possible to track the function of genes while they are active. Scientists need to make pictures of the function of genes during a certain process in progress in order to identify that process well. One of the important points of laboratory investigations in the field of genomics is the use of model species.

Individual genes and their location along chromosomes may be very similar in different species; Therefore, genomic studies in a number of model species provide information that can be used for other species as well.

For example, the results obtained from the study on fruit flies or yeast are also applicable to humans. If scientists find out exactly how the body reacts to tissue transplants, they will be able to improve cell transplant and repair systems, and finally, knowing the factors that determine the amount and type of chemicals made in a cell will lead to better and new industrial biotechnology processes will make it possible. All these successes and advances are made in the shadow of benefiting from the new knowledge of genomics, and the molecular techniques used in genomics provide the possibility of studying biological systems with very high accuracy and sensitivity that could not be achieved before.

5 basic principles of nutritional genomics

- ❖ Diet can be an important risk factor for various diseases in some people under certain conditions.
- ❖ Common chemicals in the diet alter gene expression or genetic makeup (directly or indirectly).
- ❖ The effect of diet on health depends on a person's genetic makeup.
- ❖ Some genes or their variants, which may play a role in chronic diseases, are regulated by using a suitable diet.
- ❖ Dietary interventions based on knowledge of nutritional status and genotype can be used to develop an individualized diet plan focused on optimizing health as well as preventing or reducing the incidence of chronic diseases.

The relationship between genetics and personal nutrition

Since personalized nutrition is new territory in relation to genetics, it can be understood that there is still much to learn in the scientific world. So you don't have to worry about the details, you can apply some simple tips based on what has already been specified.

Properties of food sources and the importance of nutrition in genetic health

Nutrients prevent DNA damage (mutations).

The following include important nutrients to prevent mutations that can lead to major diseases such as cancer or heart disease:

➤ Carotenoids (such as: carrots, pumpkins, yellow and red peppers, tomatoes and green leafy vegetables).

➤ Vitamin E (such as: avocado, seeds and nuts).

Foods that facilitate DNA synthesis. Foods that are important for cell growth (hair, skin, nails, etc.) and fetal growth during pregnancy include:

➤ Folic acid (such as whole grains, green leafy vegetables, legumes and citrus fruits).

➤ Vitamin B12 (such as: eggs, seafood, fish and meat).

➤ Zinc (such as: wheat germ, pumpkin seeds, nuts).

➤ Magnesium (such as cocoa found in dark chocolate, bananas, avocados).

Foods that repair DNA. They are very important nutrients for DNA mutation repair in our body including:

➤ Vitamin B3 or niacin (such as: peanuts, sunflower seeds, mushrooms and chicken).

➤ Folic acid (such as: leafy vegetables, enriched grains and fruits).

It has been noted that different types of food provide beneficial properties for genetic health. It should also be noted that the group of foods consists not only of nutrients, but also of antioxidants, polyphenols, biologically active molecules, etc.

5 basic principles of nutritional genomics

* ❖ Diet can be an important risk factor for various diseases in some people under certain conditions.
* ❖ Common chemicals in the diet alter gene expression or genetic makeup (directly or indirectly).
* ❖ The effect of diet on health depends on a person's genetic makeup.
* ❖ Some genes or their variants, which may play a role in chronic diseases, are regulated by using a suitable diet.
* ❖ Dietary interventions based on knowledge of nutritional status and genotype can be used to develop an individualized diet plan focused on optimizing health as well as preventing or reducing the incidence of chronic diseases.

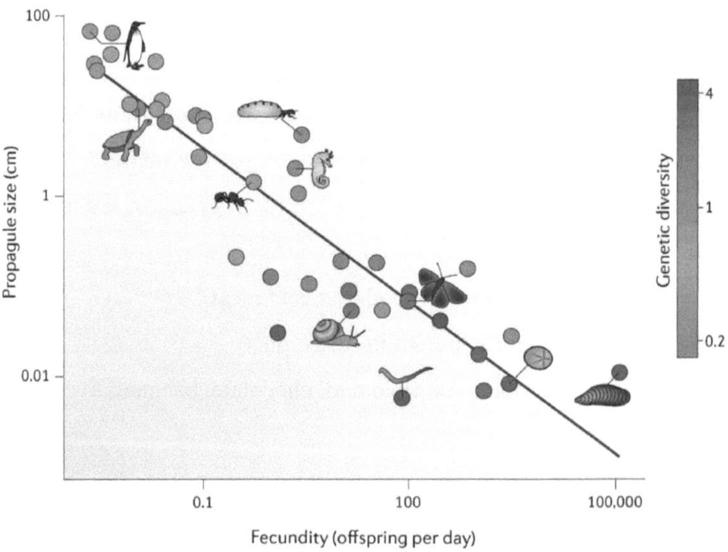

Figure 32. Determinants of genetic diversity

The relationship between genetics and personal nutrition

Since personalized nutrition is new territory in relation to genetics, it can be understood that there is still much to learn in the scientific world. So you don't have to worry about the details. You can apply some simple tips based on what has already been specified.

The relationship between intelligence, brain structure and genes

During human evolution, our brains have developed a lot. One of the areas that has developed over the last few million years is the cerebral cortex. This area processes sensory information and leads to movement and is responsible for our higher level functions such as language processing and problem solving. Scientists focus on the structure of the cerebral cortex and discuss the reasons for its evolution throughout our lives and our evolution as a species to understand where heredity interacts with our intelligence.

New research on hundreds of developing brains showed the existence of a combination in certain areas of the cerebral cortex that develops from childhood to adulthood and is enhanced during adulthood and is related to heredity. They found surface area in areas related to intelligence.

The surface area of the brain shows the interaction between brain genes, intelligence and development. An analysis on the brains of 600 children shows a connection between the surface area of the brain and heritability in important areas of the brain for cognition.

During human evolution, our brains have become very large. One of these important areas that is highly developed is the cerebral cortex. The researchers also found a genetic link between IQ test scores and the surface area associated with intelligence, and this was published in the journal Neuroscience.

"I think it's a big deal," said neuroscientist Rachel Brower at the University of Utrecht in the Netherlands. The authors of the study identified areas of the brain where variables are largely determined by genes by examining neural connections and developmental and neurodevelopmental development. This is an attempt to link heredity with what is the broader meaning of heredity (i.e. intelligence). The authors of the article reviewed brain imaging with MRI of 677 children. The scans helped them examine the children's brains, examining the twists and turns of the cortex.

By relating brain structures and genetic variables in the samples, researchers can determine which genes organize the brain during development and growth. Using processing tools, researchers determined its cortex and cross-section.

This is a measurement as if you have removed a part of the brain and removed its folds and spread it like a pizza, says A.J. Eric Schmidt, a neurologist at the University of Pennsylvania and one of the authors of this article. Brewer says: The research results point to the importance of specific surface area in evolution, while until now it has not attracted much attention compared to the total volume and cortical thickness.

The researchers also tested the heritability of these characteristics by comparing brains in a sample that included a large number of identical and non-identical twins and family members. Based on common genes through family proximity, they were able to determine the connections between genetics and some brain characteristics.

The cross-sectional area and structure of the brain in humans' changes to a great extent, and scientists realized that the cross-sectional area of the brain is largely hereditary. Genetic factors determine 85% of the variables and this is similar to the results of previous studies.

That's a big part of changeability, says Schmidt. Genes really play a role in determining the global cross section. The scientists also found that cortical thickness and cross-sectional area of the brain were genetically related in these children, and this is contrary to previous information in adults that different genetic factors are the basis for creating cross-sectional area versus cortical thickness.

This was stated by John Gilmore, a psychiatrist at the University of North Carolina. Previously, Gilmore, Schmidt and their colleagues had investigated the genetic relationship between cortical thickness and cross-sectional area in infants. Brewer says: "If we can really figure out which genes make this connection and why they grow individually as people get older, that will really help transform our understanding of evolution." Yes, this seems like an important effect, but if we have a small or large cross section, what does this have to do with IQ?

The researchers also focused on regional differences in the brain. After dividing the cross-section of the brain into 80,000 small pieces, they were able to compare the cross-sections in different brain regions.

Cross-checking this information with genetic information allowed the researchers to determine the extent to which the differences were related to heredity. When scientists precisely calculated cross-sectional differences, they were able to see which areas of the brain were closely and deeply related to heredity and genetics. These regions, which are closely related to heredity, include narrow bands of the frontal and temporal lobes, and these are associated with language processing and intelligence. Strong brains are associated with parts of the brain that develop during development.

According to other studies, these parts are very different in non-human primates. Schmidt says: This led us to imagine that there is a genetic factor that affects all these regions, which is an evolutionary story.

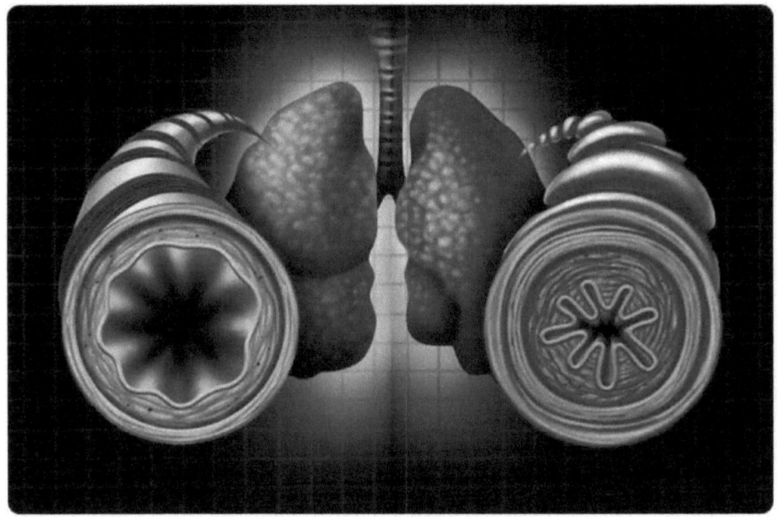

Figure 33. The Genetics of Asthma

These regions are parts that grow rapidly during childhood, and this shows that some genes that cause individual differences in humans may be things that have evolved over time. I found it very interesting, I want to know what those genes are. This study does not specify exactly which genes do this. To determine those genes, it may be necessary to take larger samples.

By analyzing descriptive brain maps, along with the results of IQ tests used on children, the researchers were able to determine which areas of the cortex are associated with higher performance in perception and may be related to heredity. Their results identified few regions, but one region, namely the left supra marginal gyrus region, remained truly associated with genetic structure, and this is the sensory and receptive language region in most people.

The correlation is the same, that is, there is a genetic overlap between IQ and cross-sectional area. This is not the first time that it shows the connection with intelligence. Schmidt says that although IQ is a useful and valuable tool, it is not a direct measure of intelligence. Genetics, education and environment, but it is not under the complete control of the size of the brain or the cross section of different parts of the brain and genes. Sometimes the shrinking of the brain size, by creating a need in the individual, leads to the development of emotional intelligence because the weak person, instead of trusting in his own abilities, tries to use the collective power and cooperation with others to solve his problems.

These results are interesting in part because not much work has been done to look at how cross-sectional relationships relate to intelligence. Most of the effects seem to be general, and there seems to be a general genetic factor that is good for your brain and intelligence, for example. However, there is a positive impression about the study and its findings. The significance of the obtained results for the relationship between brain structure and intelligence is doubtful.

Yes, this relationship seems important. But if the sample level and cross-sectional area under investigation is larger or smaller, how will the communication with IQ be? He says that this causes scientists to see a connection between the structure of the brain, but although others have expressed such a connection, there are also those who have not done so, and the connection is weak in adults.

Schmidt explains that the foundation of intelligence is a sensitive issue in neuroscience. He says: I imagine what stimulates our mental abilities. It is one of the basic questions in neuroscience and it is one of the issues that made me interested in neuroscience. Why do we have something that takes so much energy from us? This article will definitely have many benefits for us. The role of genes in the development of the brain, which is completely directional and specific, proves the purposefulness of the genetic map even beyond the sudden development of the brain size in the last two million years.

The development of the brain of human ancestors in the last two million years is a sudden and evolutionary leap that shows the law and program in the gene program, and this law that sometimes causes the speed of development and enlargement of the brain in a period suddenly increases and sometimes slows down.

Sometimes it declines and enters a return course, it indicates the lawfulness and purposefulness of the gene map. Beyond this view, new discoveries show that the development of brain size is not a general and random and blind flow, but this development is in the direction of the development of a specific part of the brain related to language perception and understanding (linguistic understanding is only limited to understanding words and It is not the common languages of the world, but a deeper concept that means understanding the meanings and intentions of events and currents and reaching from details to generalities and abstract thinking...; That is, this particular part of the brain develops during a previous program and independently of thousands of other parts of the brain.

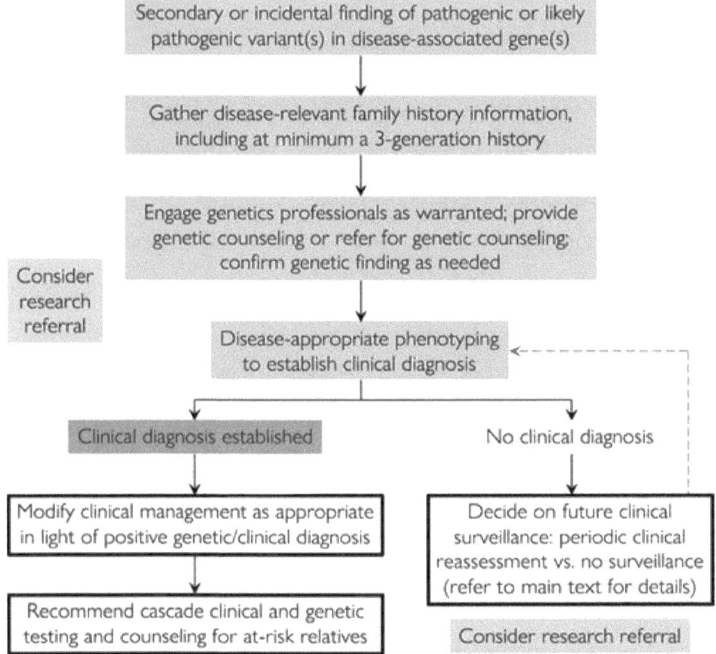

Figure 34. Genetic Testing for Inherited Cardiovascular Diseases

If among thousands of choices, and thousands of choices, only one of the choices is repeated many times, a wise person will not think that this repetition was created during a blind and random process.

Yards of life of the earth is not possible blindly and randomly (for the formation of a simple chain of 32 amino acids of protein, more than ten to the power of 41 tests should be performed so that the possibility of the formation of this protein chain is possible. Each hour is 3600 seconds, each day is 84600 seconds, and a year is 31536000 seconds, which means approximately 3 x 10 to the power of seven.

How many seconds are there in a billion years?

Approximately 3 x 10 to the power of sixteen. And in thirteen billion years, about 4 x 10 to the power of seventeen. If one test is performed every second, the total number of tests in these thirteen billion years will be approximately 4 x 10 to the seventeenth power which is much less than the tests required to form a protein chain with 32 amino acids.

It means that there is absolutely no possibility of random formation of even a chain of 32 amino acids in the entire life of the universe, let alone the life of the earth. How is the complex organization of the brain structure possible with millions of random protein chains and fat and carbohydrate chains?

And while the structure of the brain is not a fixed and inflexible structure, it can constantly change under the influence of genes and environmental changes and with complex systems such as inter-neuron communication! Why a large group of people today have reached this conclusion that creation is random is related to them!

Smart people should thank their mothers because basically mothers are the agents of transferring intelligence genes. And it is necessary for men to consider intelligence as a fundamental part of women's attractiveness. (Scientists have come to the conclusion that the higher a woman's intelligence is, the less attractive she is to men.) This idea is basically conditional genes. It is known as conditioned gene. (These genes are genes that are used in different ways) and these genes have a kind of biochemical sign that allows searching for its origin and root.

(Conditional genes are genes that are activated only if they are passed from one of the parents. For example, genes related to intelligence seem to be activated only when they are inherited from the mother) and what is noteworthy is that some of these Genes can function only when they come from the mother's side, and if they come from the father's side, they do not show activity, and thus there are other genes that are not functional except when they come from the father's side, and if it is from the mother's side, the action will be stopped.

The mother's genes go directly to the cerebral cortex, while the father's genes enter the limbic system. We know that intelligence has a hereditary aspect, but even in the past, we thought that many aspects of intelligence are jointly inherited from parents.

But a number of studies show that children inherit intelligence from their mothers because intelligence genes are on X chromosomes. The first study in this case was done in Cambridge University in 1984 and many other studies were done after that.

In these studies, the joint evolution of the brain and the quality of the genome were analyzed and they concluded that mother's genes are more effective than other genes in the development of thinking centers in the brain. In the first experiment, the researchers took mouse embryos from the genes of the father or mother. But when it was time to transfer them to the mother's mouse uterus, the embryos died.

Here we have an egg cell that contains the complete chromosomes of an asexual cell instead of a combination of sperm and egg. Then, with stimulation, this egg cell is forced to multiply and then it becomes a complete organism, which is genetically completely similar to its parent.

It seems that there are conditioned genes that are active only when they are inherited from the mother, and these genes are vital for the healthy development of the fetus, and on the other hand, there are genes that are active only when they are inherited from the father and for growth. Tissues are important for the formation of membranes around the embryo.

At that time, researchers thought that these genes are important in the development of the fetus and preferably play an important role in the life of animals and humans, and maybe they perform some functions of the brain. But the problem was how to prove this opinion because the embryos formed from one of the parents die quickly.

But the researchers found a solution: they found that if protection is created against harmful and invasive embryonic cells and other cells are used, the embryos can be kept alive. With this method, a number of genetically processed mice can be saved. And surprisingly, they did not grow like normal mice.

The fetuses that were from the mother's genes had larger brains and smaller bodies. And those that were from the father's genes had small brains and large bodies. By further analyzing these differences, the researchers identified the cells that contained the father's or mother's genes in six different parts of the brain. and these cells performed different cognitive tasks such as eating habits and memory.

During the first days of fetal development, cells may appear anywhere in the brain, but with the further formation of the fetus and the continuation of its growth, paternal genes accumulate in some emotional centers in the brain such as the hypothalamus, the limbic system, the preoptic area, and the septum. These areas are part of the emotional system and are responsible for our survival and are involved in tasks such as sexual activity, food, hatred and enmity, and researchers have found traces of the father's genes in the cerebral cortex, whose task is the development of advanced cognitive responsibilities such as intelligence, thought, language, and It is planning, they did not find it.

New studies, new light on intelligence

Scholars have come to this theory: for example, Robert Lirk showed that most of a child's intelligence is based on the X chromosome, and he showed that women have two X chromosomes, so it is more likely that they carry genes related to intelligence with them. Carrying the intelligence gene does not mean that women have bigger and smarter brains.

Based on scientific studies, it has been proven that the average brain of women is less than that of men. Being a carrier of a superior gene means that this gene can be passed on to the next generations, but it does not necessarily perform its function in the carrier's own body. In the previous parts, we explained that there are many genes that are activated in certain conditions. So, being a gene carrier does not mean that gene is functioning in the body of the carrier. Recently, researchers from Ulm University in Germany investigated the genes responsible for brain destruction and found out that there are a large number of these genes that are related to cognitive power in the X chromosomes.

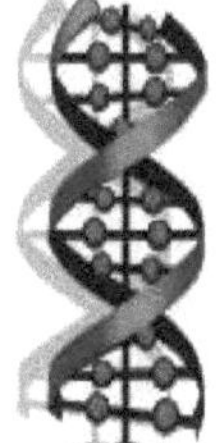

Figure 35. Genetics

A remarkable result was obtained from a large analysis in Glasgow, Scotland. In this study, 12,686 young people who were between 14 and 22 years old were investigated and the researchers took into account several factors, including: face color, the role of education in economic and social growth, and economic status, and the researchers found that the most important determinant of average intelligence is mother's intelligence. And they realized that the average intelligence of young people is fifteen degrees different from the intelligence of their mothers.

Genes are not the only factor

From the side of genes, we can see other studies that show that the mother plays an important role in the intellectual development of the child through physical and emotional connection. In fact, studies show that the secure connection between the mother and the child is prominently related to intelligence.

Researchers from the University of Minnesota found that children who developed strong relationships between themselves and their mothers were better able to learn complex puzzles, and these children were more stable and less likely to fail in solving problems.

Because this strong connection gave children the necessary security to explore the world and confidence in solving problems without losing their personality.

In addition, mothers are interested in giving their children the highest level of support to solve problems, and this helps to increase their abilities, and researchers at the University of Washington have clarified the importance of emotional connection for brain development and discovered for the first time that communication with mother and mother's love is important for the development of some brain components and scientists analyzed the way a mother communicates with her children for seven years and understood that when the mother is emotionally supportive of the child and the intellectual and emotional needs of the child The hippocampus in children is ten percent larger than children who were emotionally distant from their mothers.

And the hippocampus of the brain is related to memory and the ability to respond to mental pressure. This does not mean to reduce the importance of the relationship with the father, but the reason for this is the social structure that causes certain forms of growth and development in both sexes. This role difference between the two sexes is always present and it is usually the mother who spends most of her time with the child.

Can we talk about hereditary intelligence?

In fact, most of the measurements show that hereditary intelligence is between 40 and 60%, and this means that the remaining ratio is based on many factors, including living environment, motivation, and personality traits.

Intelligence is the power to solve problems and it is surprising that the limbic system plays an important role in solving problems, even if it is a simple physics or math problem, because the brain acts like a single organ, and in this way, intelligence has a deep connection with the power of rational thinking and the speed of thinking and emotions are affected.

In addition, we must not forget that even if the child's IQ is high, it is necessary for the child to stimulate that intelligence throughout his life, because if the intelligence is not stimulated with new stimuli, it will gradually decline, and despite the effects of genes, it is worthy of fathers. Encourage them to contribute to the education of children, especially from the emotional aspect. The intelligence with which we are born is important, but it is not certain and fixed.

The effect of genetics on obesity and overweight

The effect of genetics on obesity: changes in the BNDF gene cause people to have a greater desire to eat high-fat foods and in large portions. In addition, these people are prone to obesity again after following a slimming diet. Therefore, they should continue their slimming diets and exercise in the long term so as not to gain weight again.

Other tests that are recommended for obese people:
- Genetic panel of susceptibility to diabetes.
- Genetic panel of forgetfulness and mental disorders (Alzheimer-Parkinson).
- Appetite genetic panel.

The effect of genetics on weight fitness

Fat metabolism in the body is related to genetics. In fact, there is no direct relationship between diet and body weight. This means that some people consume a lot of food.

But their weight does not increase in relation to the food consumed, while some people gain a lot of weight by eating little food. This difference is due to the effect of genetics on weight ratio.

There is no doubt that diet and physical activity both play an important role in determining our weight. But according to recent studies, the cause of 40-70% of obesity cases is genetic. It has even been determined that the response of obese people to slimming diets with various sports also differs from each other. In other words, genes (inheritance) affect how people absorb, metabolize and store fat in their bodies. Therefore, a person may become fat by eating a certain food.

What is the importance of genetic testing in the treatment of obesity?

By performing special tests on each person's DNA, it is possible to find out whether he carries certain genes that make him prone to overweight and obesity. Also, what type of diet and which group of sports can overcome obesity or overweight problems? A person will find out how much his obesity has a genetic background. If obesity has genetic roots, the doctor can choose the best treatment method by finding out which of the individual's genes are involved.

The diet is different for each of the genes. When a person is not aware of his genetic obesity, he may choose a diet that not only does not cause weight loss but also aggravates the person's obesity. A person will find out whether physical activity and exercise are effective in losing weight or not. And which exercise should be done for his fitness. The doctor can easily determine whether the drug treatment is useful for the person or not. The genes studied in the special test for the study of genes related to weigh proportionality of 6 genes related to obesity are studied.

What is molecular genetic testing?

According to studies, changes in the FABP2 gene cause abdominal fat and resting metabolism. These people should avoid consuming saturated fatty acids and use more unsaturated fatty acids (especially omega-3) (Mediterranean diet). In addition, the consumption of complex carbohydrates (found in vegetables, bread and whole grains) will also help in fat metabolism and increase insulin sensitivity.

Autosomal dominant inheritance pattern

The autosomal dominant trait has two specific characteristics. First, the one that is transmitted through asexual chromosomes, and the other one that manifests itself in the heterozygous state (a healthy gene copy + a defective gene copy).

In this case, if one of the parents has a dominant trait or disease, all his children have a 50% chance of inheriting that trait or disease. Examples of these diseases are Marfan, Huntington, muscular dystrophy and... These diseases have variable severity. In other words, clinical symptoms in different people can be different from one person to another. For example, in polycystic kidney disease, during which the kidney has multiple cysts.

A person may show symptoms of the disease in early adulthood. However, another person can be without symptoms until the end of old age. The interesting thing about these diseases is that a person can look completely normal without any symptoms even though he is heterozygous. In this case, which is called reduced penetrance, over the generations, the modifying effects of other genes and the interaction of genes with the environment can prevent the occurrence of symptoms.

For example, people who have a mutated gene predisposing to breast cancer have an 80% chance of developing cancer. In other words, due to the presence of other genes, the probability of the mutation of this gene has decreased by 20%.

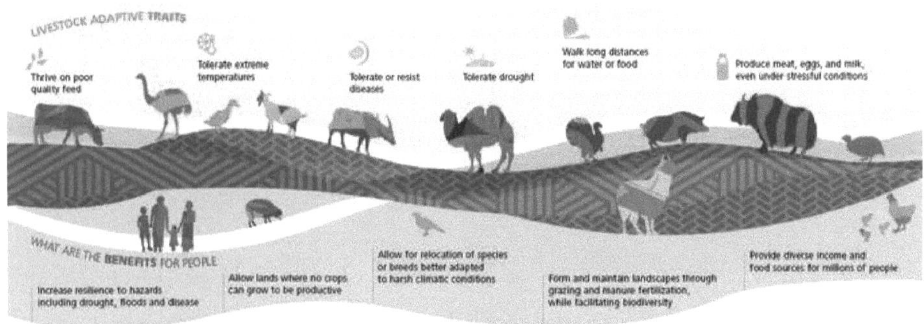

Figure 36. Animal genetics

Another interesting point is that in some people with a dominant trait, parents can lack any dominant gene. In other words, a child with a dominant disease is born from parents who are completely healthy. In this case, following an error during gene transfer, a new mutation occurs. An example of this condition is achondroplasia, in which parents have a normal height, but their child has a form of dwarfism with short arms and legs.

Regarding how to diagnose autosomal dominant disease with the help of genealogy, it should be kept in mind that sex chromosomes have no role in this disease. As a result, transmission between generations is carried out by people of both sexes, and in addition, the possibility of infection is equal between men and women. Finally, it is observed continuously in several generations in autosomal dominant diseases.

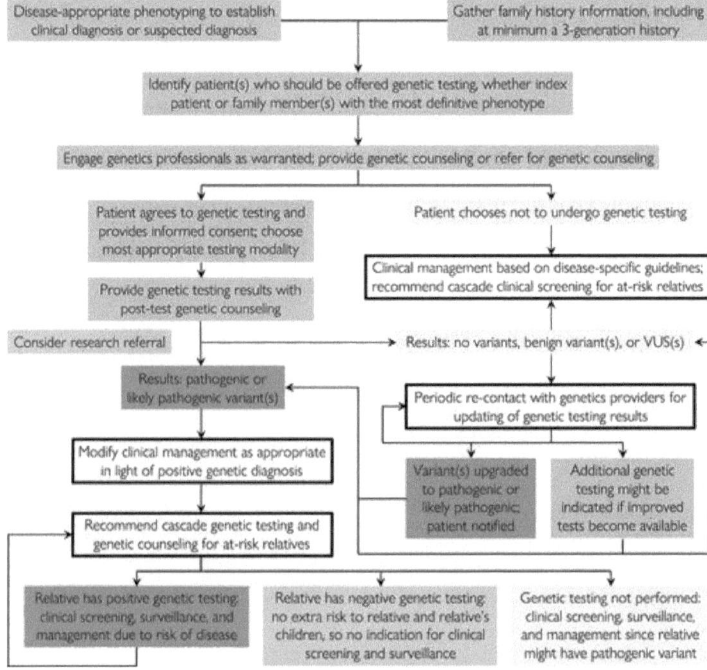

Figure 37. Genetic Testing for Inherited Cardiovascular Diseases

References

Scotto, J, Fears, T.R, Fraumeni, J.r. Solar radiation. In: Schottenfeld D, Fraumeni JF Jr, eds: Cancer Epidemiology and Prevention. 2nd Ed. New York, NY: Oxford University Press; 1996; 355-72.

Vogelstein B, Kinzler KW. Cancer genes and the pathways they control. Nat Med. 2004; 10(8): 789-99.

Vogelstein B, Fearon ER, Hamilton SR, Kern SE, et al. Genetic alterations during colorectal- tumor development. N Engl J Med. 1988; 319(9): 525-532.

Sonnenschein C, Soto AM. Theories of carcinogenesis: an emerging perspective. Semi Cancer Biol. 2008; 18(5): 372-7.

Pakin DM. The global health burden of infection-associated cancers in the years 2002. Int J Cancer.2006; 118(12): 3030-44.

National RC. Committee to Assess Health Risks from Exposure to Low Levels of Inoizing Radiation: BEIR VII Phase 2. Washington. 2011.

Fazel R, Krumholz HM, Wang R, et al. Exposure to Low-dose ionizing radiation from medical imaging procedures. N Engl J Med. 2009; 361(9): 849-57.

William WN Jr, Heymach JV, Kim ES, et al. Molecular targets for cancer chemoprevention. Nat Rev Drug Discov. 2009; 8(3): 213-25.

Seto M, Honma K, Nakagawa M. Diversity of genome profiles in malignant lymphoma. Cancer Science. 2010; 101: 573-578.

Staal SP, Huebner k, Croce CM, Parsa N, et al. The akt-1 proto oncogene maps to human chromosome 14, band q32, a site of chromosome rearrangement in some hematopoietic neo plasma. Journal of Genomics. 1988; 2: 96-98.

Park M, Testa JR, Blair DG, Parsa N, et al. Two rearranged Met alleles on chromosome 7 to other markers tightly linked to cystic fibrosis. Proceeding of the National Academy of Sciences, USA. 1988; 85: 2667-2671.

Offit K, Parsa N, Jhanwar SC, Filippa DA, et al. (9;14) (p13;q32): Denotes a subset of low to intermediate grade B-cell Non-Hodgkin's lymphoma. Journal of the American Society of Hematology(Blood). 1992; 80:45-60.

Parsa N, Gaidano G, Mukherjee AB, Hauptschein RS, et al. Cytogenetic and molecular analysis of 6q deletions in Burkitt's lymphoma cell lines. Journal of Genes, Chromosomes & Cancer. 1994; 9(1): 13-18.

Papanicolaou GJ, Parsa N, Meltzer PS, Trent JM. Assignments of interferon gama receptor(INFGR1) to human chromosome bands 6q24.1→q 24.2 by Fluorescent in Situ hybridization. Journal of Cytogenetics and Cell Genetics. 1997; 76: 181-182.

Cigudosa JC, Parsa N, Louie DC, Filippa DA, et al. Cytogenetic analysis of 363 consecutively ascertained diffuse large B-cell lymphomas. Journal of Genes, chromosoma & Cancer. 1999; 25: 123-133.

Shtivelman E, Lifshitz B, Gale RP, Canaani E. Fused transcript of abl and bcr genes in chronic myelogenous leukemia. Nature. 1985; 315: 550-554.

Druker BJ, Talpaz M, Resta DJ, et al. Efficacy and safety of a specific inhibitor of the BCR-ABL tyrosine kinase in chronic myeloid leukemia. N Engl J Med. 2001; 344: 1031-1037.

Joensuu H, Dimitrijevic S. Tyrosine kinase inhibitor imatinib (STI571) as an anticancer agent for solid tumors. Ann Med. 2001; 33: 451-455.

King CR, Kraus MH, Aaronson SA. Amplification of a novel v-erbB-related gene in a human mammary carcinoma. Science. 1985; 229: 974-976.

Heinrich MC, Blanke CD, Druker BJ, Corless CL. Inhibition of KIT tyrosine kinase activity: a novel molecular approach to the treatment of KIT-positive malignancies. J Clin Oncol. 2002; 20: 1692-1703.

Thomas RK, et al. High-throuphut oncogene mutation profiling in human cancer. Nature Genetics. 2007; 39: 347-351.

Weinstein IB, Joe AK. Mechanisms of disease: Oncogene addiction-arationale for molecular targeting in cancer theraphy. Nature Clinical Practice Oncology. 2006; 3: 448-457.

Qingyi W, Li L, Chen D. DNA Repair, Genetic Instability, and Cancer. World Scientific. ISBN. 2007; 981-270-014-5.

Hogervorst FB, et al. "Large genomic deletions and duplications in the BRCA1 gene identified by a novel quantitative method". Cancer Res. 2003; 63 (7): 1449–1453.

Friedenson B. "A theory that explains the tissue specificity of BRCA1/2 related and other hereditary cancers". Journal of Medicine and Medical Sciences. 2010; 1 (8): 372–384.

Tonin PN, Serova O, Lenoir G, Lynch H, et al. "BRCA1 mutations in Ashkenazi Jewish women". American Journal of Human Genetics. 1995; 57 (1): 189.

Narod SA, Foulkes WD. "BRCA1 and BRCA2: 1994 and beyond". Nature Reviews on Cancer. 2004; 4 (9): 665–676.

Wei Q, Lei L, Chen D. DNA Repair, Genetic Instability and cancer. World scientific. 2007; 270-014.

Fesik SW, Shi Y. "Controlling the caspases". Science. 2001; 294 (5546): 1477–1478.

Murphy KM, Ranganathan V, Farnsworth ML, Kavallaris M, et al. "Bcl-2 inhibits Bax translocation from cytosol to mitochondria during drug-induced apoptosis of human tumor cells". Cell Death Differ. 2000; 7 (1): 102–111.

Santos A, Susin SA, Daugas E, Ravagnan L, et al. "Two Distinct Pathways Leading to Nuclear Apoptosis". Journal of Experimental Medicine. 2000; 192 (4): 571–580.

Zhou GP, Doctor K. Subcellular location prediction of apoptosis proteins. PROTEINS: Structure, Function, and Genetics. 2003; 50: 44-48.

Thompson CB. Apoptosis in the pathogenesis and treatment of disease. Science. 1995; 267(5203): 1456-62

Matlashewski G, Lamb P, Pim D, Peacock J, et al. "Isolation and characterization of a human p53 cDNA clone: expression of the human p53 gene". EMBO J. 3 (13): 3257–3262.

May P, May E. Twenty years of p53 research: structural and functional aspects of the p53 protein. Oncogene. 1999; 18: 7621–7636.

McBride OW, Merry D, Givol D. "The gene for human p53 cellular tumor antigen is located on chromosome 17 short arm (17p13)". Proc. Natl. Acad. Sci. U.S.A. 1986; 83 (1): 130–134.

Isobe M, Emanuel BS, Givol D, Oren M, Croce CM. "Localization of gene for human p53 tumor antigen to band 17p13". Nature. 1986; 320 (6057): 84–85.

Hollstein M, Sidransky D, Vogelstein B, Harris CC. "p53 mutations in human cancers". Science. 1991; 253 (5015): 49–53.

Baak JP, Path FR, Hermsen MA, Meijer G, et al. Genomics and proteomics in cancer. Eur J Cancer. 2003; 39: 1199-1215.

Scarpa A, Moore PS, Rigaud G, Meenestrina F. Genetic in primary mediastinal B-cell lymphoma: an updata. Leukemia & Lymphoma. 2001; 411(2): 47-53.

Collins F. The human genome project and beyond. US-Department of energy. 2003; 3.

Pollak JR, Perou CM, Alizadeh AA, Eisen MB, et al. Genome-wide analysis of DNA copy-number changes using Cdna microarrays. Nature Genet. 2003; 23: 41-46.

Kashiwagi H, Uchida K. Genome- wide profiling of gene amplification and deletion in cancer. Human Cell. 2003; 13: 135-141.

Albertson DG, Pinkel D. Genomic microarrays in human genetic disease and cancer. Hum Mol Genet. 2003; 12: 145-52.

Mohr S, Leikauf GD, Keith G, Rihn BH. Microarrays as cancer keys: an array of possibilities. J Clin Oncology. 2002; 20: 3165-3175.

Tachdjian G, Aboura A, Lapierre JM, Viguei F. Cytogenetic analysis from DNA by comparative genomic hybridization. Ann Genet. 2002; 43: 147-154.

Bhagwan ‹Bhagwan; Sharma ‹R.K. (January 1٢٠٠٩ ‹). *Charaka Samhita*. Chowkhamba Sanskrit Series.

Zirkle C (1941). "Natural Selection before the "Origin of Species"". *Proceedings of the American Philosophical Society* ٨۴ (۱): ٧١–١٢٣.

Cosman ‹Madeleine Pelner; Jones ‹Linda Gale. *Handbook to life in the medieval world*. Infobase Publishing. pp. 528–529.

HaLevi ‹Judah ‹translated and annotated by N. Daniel Korobkin. *The Kuzari: In Defense of the Despised Faith*‹ p. 38 ‹I:95: "This phenomenon is common in genetics as well—often we find a son who does not resemble his father at all ‹but closely resembles his grandfather. Undoubtedly ‹the genetics and resemblance were dormant within the father even though they were not outwardly apparent.

Bateson ‹William (1907). "The Progress of Genetic Research". In Wilks ‹W. (editor). *Report of the Third 1906 International Conference on Genetics: Hybridization (the cross-breeding of genera or species)‹ the cross-breeding of varieties‹ and general plant breeding*. London: Royal Horticultural Society.

Beadle GW ‹Tatum EL. Genetic Control of Biochemical Reactions in Neurospora. Proc Natl Acad Sci U S A. 1941 Nov 15;27(11):499-506.

Luria SE. Reactivation of Irradiated Bacteriophage by Transfer of Self-Reproducing Units. Proc Natl Acad Sci U S A. 1947 Sep;33(9):253-64.

Bernstein C. Deoxyribonucleic acid repair in bacteriophage. Microbiol Rev. 1981 Mar;45(1):72-98.

Watson JD ‹Crick FH (Apr 1953). "Molecular structure of nucleic acids; a structure for deoxyribose nucleic acid". *Nature* ١٧١ (٤٣٥٦): ٧٣٧–٨.

Jacob F1 ‹Perrin D ‹Sánchez C‹ Monod J ‹Edelstein S. [The operon: a group of genes with expression coordinated by an operator. C.R.Acad. Sci. Paris 250 (1960) 1727-1729].

Min Jou W ‹Haegeman G ‹Ysebaert M ‹Fiers W (May 1972). "Nucleotide sequence of the gene coding for the bacteriophage MS2 coat protein". *Nature* ٢٣٧ (٥٣٥٠): ٨٢–٨.

Fiers W ‹Contreras R ‹Duerinck F ‹Haegeman G ‹Iserentant D ‹Merregaert J ‹ Min Jou W ‹Molemans F et al. (1976). "Complete nucleotide-sequence of bacteriophage MS2-RNA – primary and secondary structure of replicase gene". *Nature* ۲۶۰ (۵۵۵۱): ۵۰۰–۵۰۷.

Sanger F ،Air GM ،Barrell BG، Brown NL ،Coulson AR ،Fiddes CA ،Hutchison CA ،Slocombe PM ،Smith M et al. (Feb 1977). "Nucleotide sequence of bacteriophage phi X174 DNA". *Nature* ۲۶۵ (۵۵۹۶): ۶۸۷–۹۵.

Kerem B; Rommens JM; Buchanan JA; Markiewicz; Cox; Chakravarti; Buchwald; Tsui (September 1989).

Fleischmann RD; Adams MD; White O; Clayton; Kirkness; Kerlavage; Bult; Tomb; Dougherty; Merrick; McKenney; Sutton; Fitzhugh; Fields; Gocyne; Scott; Shirley; Liu; Glodek; Kelley; Weidman; Phillips; Spriggs; Hedblom; Cotton; Utterback; Hanna; Nguyen; Saudek et al. (July 1995).

Giovannucci Edward. Nutrient and Gene Interactions in Cancer,Chapter 1. Edited by: Sang-Woon Choi, Simonetta Friso. In: Nutrient-gene interactions in cancer. CRC Press, Taylor & Francis Group. 2006; 1-17.

Friso S, Choi S.W. Gene-Nutrient Interactions in One-Carbon Metabolism. Current Drug Metabolism. 2005; 6 (1): 37-46.

Wai-Nang P. Lee and Vay Liang W.Go. Nutrient-Gene Interaction: Tracer-Based Metabolomics. J. Nutr. 2005; 135: 3027S–32S, .

Ramezani A, Koohdani F, et al. Effects of administration of omega-3 fatty acids with or without vitamin E supplementation on adiponectin gene expression in PBMCs and serum adiponectin and adipocyte fatty acid-binding protein levels in male patients with CAD. growth. 2015; 8:11-3.

Ramezani A, Djazayeri A, et al. omega-3 fatty acids/vitamin e behave synergistically on adiponectin receptor-1 and adiponectin receptor-2 gene expressions in peripheral blood mononuclear cell of coronary artery disease patients. Current Topics in Nutraceutical Research. 2015;13(2):23-32.

Yousefinejad A, Siassi F, et al. Effect of Genistein and L-Carnitine and Their Combination on Gene Expression of Hepatocyte HMG-COA Reductase and LDL Receptor in Experimental Nephrotic Syndrome. Iranian journal of public health. 2015;44(10):1339-1347.

Ramezani, A. Djalali M. Effects of administration of omega-3 fatty acids with or without vitamin E supplementation on adiponectin gene expression in PBMCs and serum adiponectin and adipocyte fatty acid-binding protein levels in male patients with CAD. growth, 2015; 8: 11-13.

Ramezani, A., et al., omega-3 fatty acids/vitamin e behave synergistically on adiponectin receptor-1 and adiponectin receptor-2 gene expressions in peripheral blood mononuclear cell of coronary artery disease patients. Current Topics In Nutraceutical Research, 2015; 13(2):23-32.

Ham M-S, Lee J-K, et al. S-adenosyl methionine specifically protects the anticancer effect of 5-FU via DNMTs expression in human A549 lung cancer cells. Molecular and clinical oncology. 2013;1(2):373-378.

Rowland GW, Schwartz GG, et al. Calcium Intake and Prostate Cancer Among African Americans: Effect Modification by Vitamin D Receptor Calcium Absorption Genotype. J Bone Miner Res. 2012; 27(1): 187–194.

Farid E. Ahmed. Gene-Gene, Gene-Environment & Multiple Interactions in Colorectal Cancer. J Environ Sci Health C Environ Carcinog Ecotoxicol Rev.2006; 24:1-101.

Suh J, Herbig A, et al. New perspectives on folate catabolism. Annu Rev Nutr. 2001; 21:255–282.

Shane B, Stokstad E. The interrelationships among folate, vitamin B12, and methionine metabolism. Adv Nutr Res. 1983;5:133–170.

Yousefinejad A, Siassi F, et al. Effect of Genistein and L-Carnitine and Their Combination on Gene Expression of Hepatocyte HMG-COA Reductase and LDL Receptor in Experimental Nephrotic Syndrome. Iranian journal of public health. 2015;44(10):1339-1347.

Ramezani, A. Djalali M. Effects of administration of omega-3 fatty acids with or without vitamin E supplementation on adiponectin gene expression in

PBMCs and serum adiponectin and adipocyte fatty acid-binding protein levels in male patients with CAD. growth, 2015; 8: 11-13.

Ramezani, A., et al., omega-3 fatty acids/vitamin e behave synergistically on adiponectin receptor-1 and adiponectin receptor-2 gene expressions in peripheral blood mononuclear cell of coronary artery disease patients. Current Topics in Nutraceutical Research, 2015; 13(2):23-32.

Staal SP, Huebner k, Croce CM, Parsa N, et al. The akt-1 proto-oncogene maps to human chromosome 14, band q32, a site of chromosome rearrangement in some hematopoietic neoplasma. Journal of Genomics. 1988; 2: 96-98.

Park M, Testa JR, Blair DG, Parsa N, et al. Two rearranged Met alleles on chromosome 7 to other

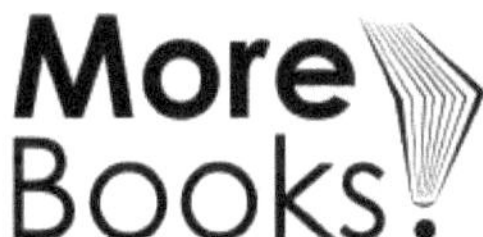

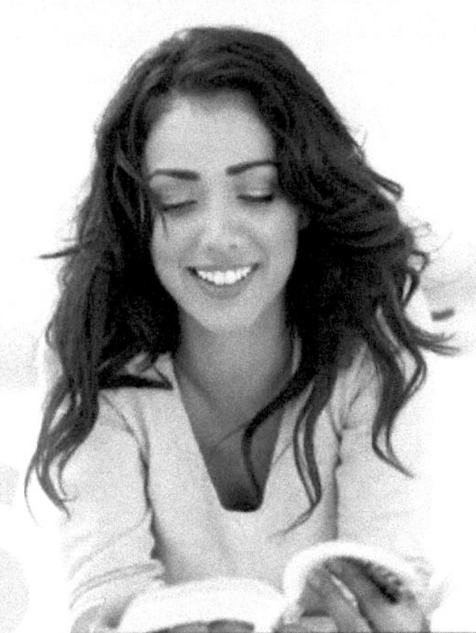

I want morebooks!

Buy your books fast and straightforward online - at one of world's fastest growing online book stores! Environmentally sound due to Print-on-Demand technologies.

Buy your books online at
www.morebooks.shop

Kaufen Sie Ihre Bücher schnell und unkompliziert online – auf einer der am schnellsten wachsenden Buchhandelsplattformen weltweit! Dank Print-On-Demand umwelt- und ressourcenschonend produziert.

Bücher schneller online kaufen
www.morebooks.shop

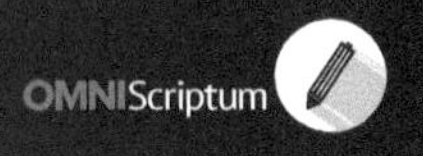

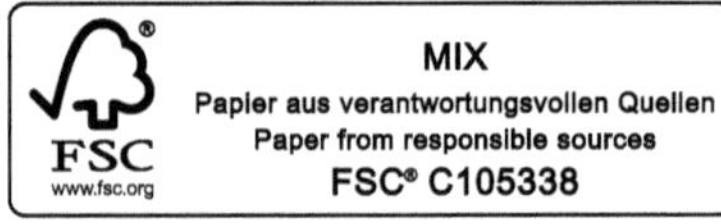

Printed by Books on Demand GmbH, Norderstedt / Germany